Empower Your Health

Empower Your Health

Optimize Your Immune System for Vibrant Health and Wellness

Lucia Cagnes, MD

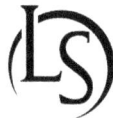

LEON SMITH
PUBLISHING

ISBN: 978-1-957972-14-5

*This transformative book is dedicated to those affected
by Human Papillomavirus (HPV), offering
a beacon of hope and knowledge.*

*It is also a tribute to the tireless medical providers
who stand by their side in this journey.*

PRAISE FOR
EMPOWER YOUR HEALTH

"*Empower Your Health* is a valuable resource providing a holistic approach for healthcare professionals. Dr. Lucia Cagnes has a deep understanding of HPV, immune health, and disease prevention. Her book offers evidence-based insights and strategies that enhance patient care and empowers individuals to take charge of their health."

~Dr. Randy Kamen
Psychologist, Coach, and Educator
Author of *Behind the Therapy Door:*
Simple Strategies to Transform Your Life

"In *Empower Your Health*, Dr. Lucia Cagnes delivers a timely and uplifting message: true wellness is within our reach—and it begins with the choices we make each day. With compassion, clarity, and the wisdom of experience, she illustrates how physical, emotional, and spiritual well-being are rooted in intentional, mindful living. From nourishing our bodies to cultivating positive thoughts and embracing the simple power of a smile, Dr. Cagnes offers both inspiration and practical guidance. This book is an essential read for anyone seeking to take control of their health, find joy from within, and build a more vibrant, connected life."

~ Julie Clarke
Co-Founder and Managing Member of For Healthy Cells
Certified Nutritional Consultant
Licensed Phlebotomist

CONTENTS

SECTION III
OPTIMIZE YOUR IMMUNE SYSTEM
FOR BETTER HEALTH

ACKNOWLEDGMENTS

First and foremost, I extend my heartfelt thanks to Peter for enlightening me on the urgency of addressing HPV not only for women but also for men. His personal experience became the catalyst for writing this book, inspiring me to offer guidance and knowledge to those who seek a better understanding of this important health condition.

I also want to take a moment to acknowledge myself for the perseverance and discipline required to complete this book—a demanding journey that has taken countless hours away from personal and family time yet has been one of the most rewarding experiences of my life.

My deepest gratitude goes to Maggie, whose meticulous editing work has brought this book to life. Without her expertise, this project would not have become the reality it is today.

I am profoundly thankful to my dedicated staff, who recognized the importance of this project and graciously adjusted my work schedule, allowing me the time and space to fully immerse myself in the creative process of writing.

To my beloved children, Jack and Charlie, thank you for your unconditional love and unwavering support. Your belief in me has kept me going.

Lastly, a special thank you to my patients. Your incredible support and encouragement throughout this process have been a constant source of motivation. You are the reason this book exists.

PREFACE

As a medical provider, I have become sensitized to the serious health-related complications of contracting an infection with HPV through my interpersonal and professional path.

I lived the struggle of my partner who, a few years ago, was dealing with life-threatening HPV-induced cancer.

Given my personal involvement as a partner in a relationship and my ongoing experience in addressing HPV-related health issues in my clinical practice, I've made the choice to impart my personal and professional insights and expertise to my readers.

Within the pages of this book, I articulate the significance of maintaining a robust and resilient immune system, emphasizing its pivotal role not just in enhancing disease prevention and combat but also in retarding the overall aging process. Additionally, I offer valuable insights to equip my readers with practical knowledge on how to achieve this goal.

Over the course of my four-decade-long medical career, I have learned and systemically organized a wealth of pertinent scientific information and knowledge that I am eager to impart to my patients, family, friends, and now, my readers.

By providing comprehensive information on the importance of early cancer diagnosis, effective screening methods, and cancer prevention strategies, this publication aims to empower individuals, healthcare professionals, and communities to take proactive steps in the fight against cancer. Together, we can enhance awareness, save lives, and work toward a future free from the burden of this devastating disease.

I trust that this publication will serve as a valuable source of information, addressing not only the issue of the HPV epidemic but also emphasizing the critical aspects of maintaining overall bodily health and disease prevention through a strong emphasis on preventive care.

I hold the belief that disseminating greater knowledge and awareness regarding the HPV epidemic will contribute to the creation of a more improved world for both our present generation and those that follow.

INTRODUCTION

I had the privilege of being born and raised in a quaint town nestled in the southern region of the picturesque and sun-kissed land of Sicily, Italy. I graduated in 1981 from medical school summa cum laude at the University of Palermo. I completed my first residency in Obstetrics and Gynecology (OB/GYN) in 1985.

In 1988, I had a blind date with the person who would later become my husband. He was a U.S. Air Force officer stationed in a NATO base located close to my hometown. There was a mutual and deep attraction from the very beginning. We developed an interest in each other and felt the need to deepen our friendship, so we began dating. We continued our relationship even after he was given a different assignment back to the U.S.

We embarked on a journey to explore some of the most breathtaking destinations on Earth. We immersed ourselves in the wonders of the world, creating treasured memories in places of awe-inspiring beauty. We wandered hand in hand through the enchanting streets of Edinburgh, indulging in the city's romantic ambiance while exploring his Scottish family's roots. We strolled along pristine beaches in Malta, our footsteps leaving imprints on the soft sand as we gazed at the crystal-clear turquoise waters. As our love deepened, so did our appreciation for the world's wonders, and we cherished every moment spent together in these extraordinary places.

He asked me to marry him before our one-year anniversary.

The Omen

I was the head assistant of the Department of OB/GYN in a small community hospital in Santhia, in the north of Italy—a small rural town located between Milan and Turin in the Pianura Padana, surrounded by rice fields.

After deciding to tie the knot, I searched for the perfect wedding gown and was able to find a beautiful dress crafted in a simple style that fit my body like a glove. I was truly excited to wear it on my special day.

I carefully packed the dress in a suitcase to travel on a ferry back to Sicily, where I would join my family and get ready for the big event in New York City. My father bought a business class ticket for me on a TWA flight, and I left Sicily from the airport in Catania.

Upon my arrival at JFK airport, I found out that the suitcase with my wedding gown was missing and never made it to its destination. My wedding day was only a few days down the road, and I would not have a wedding dress to wear.

At my wit's end, feeling utterly stressed and frustrated, I resolved to return to Sicily and call off the wedding if I couldn't find my suitcase with my wedding gown. After several frantic trips to the two major airports serving New York City, LaGuardia and JFK, I was randomly able to spot my precious suitcase on the lost and found pile, looking so sad and lonely. It had been sent to an airport in Toronto where nobody claimed it. Therefore, due to some strange combination of events, it was delivered to LaGuardia.

I thought to myself upon recovering my wedding dress at last: *This is the sign from the Universe that I am supposed to marry this man!*

Our wedding took place at the military base of Fort Hamilton in Bay Ridge, New York, on a beautiful day in October 1989.

Looking at the Verrazano-Narrows Bridge which connected Staten Island to Manhattan in the distance, I felt so much appreciation for this amazing new life that was ready to unfold for me. I was sharing a strong love with the man I chose to live with for the rest of my life in a new reality so totally different from what I was used to.

A true rollercoaster of feelings and emotions was going through me. I was excited and happy beyond words, but I was also very sad to leave my original family, friends, and my workplace behind.

A few weeks later, I found out that I was expecting my first child. Exactly nine months since my honeymoon, my baby boy was born in the West Point military hospital after a long labor. The birth of my first child motivated me to resume my medical career, interrupted because of my move to the United States. I went to school to perfect my knowledge of the English language. I took and passed my medical boards to have access to a residency program in the U.S.

My brand-new medical career took off in 1992, when I was accepted into a family practice residency program in Cincinnati, Ohio. I found out the hard way how difficult it was for a foreign doctor to be accepted in an OB/GYN residency, especially one considered to be very competitive. Being in the family practice residency had given me the advantage I needed to have access to the residency program of my choice.

I was committed to become an OB/GYN in the United States, and my perseverance came to fruition when, in 1994, I was accepted into a second year of a residency program in upstate New York. I graduated from the program in 1997, and I achieved my board certification in 1999.

After my residency, I was granted a position of clinical instructor in the Department of OB/GYN at Vanderbilt University in Nashville, Tennessee.

My dream and highest aspirations were to practice gynecology and surgery. I was never really interested in delivering babies, which is a very natural process that seldom requires any medical intervention. The chief of the OB/GYN department at Vanderbilt was not very supportive of my decision to limit my practice to GYN. I decided to resign from my position there and to find a GYN-only position in a private practice setting.

I responded to an ad of a gynecologist on Cape Cod in Massachusetts, who was nearing retirement and looking into selling his practice to a new partner. My interview was scheduled in Hyannis the day after a dreadful snowstorm in February 1999. Arriving at the airport in Providence, Rhode Island, we found the roads were totally covered in snow. There was a complete whiteout, and no lane markings or road signs were visible. The commute from the airport to our destination, a distance that typically takes about an hour and a half, took almost three hours.

The interview went well, and I was offered the new position as a partner. I was finally able to follow my passion for gynecology, surgery, infertility, and endocrinology as I envisioned.

My decision to move to Cape Cod was not an easy one, and it came with a huge price tag. I was accustomed to working in a prestigious academic environment at Vanderbilt University, a culturally stimulating place with a strong background and a leader in the field of medicine and research. The campus was beautiful and carefully arranged with a pristine landscaping design made of trees and shrubs of vibrant colors. There was an amazing library on site, and top-notch physicians and colleagues were available for consultation or referral. The short time I spent at the University represented an amazing learning experience for me. I loved the opportunity to teach medical students and residents.

We left our beautiful five-bedroom five-bathroom mansion in Brentwood, Tennessee, to move into a small, cramped country home in a very rural area of Cape Cod. The house was so small that we had to put most of our furniture into storage. My heart sank in a bucket of sorrow the moment I moved to Cape Cod and began working in a completely different environment where diversity was a remote concept.

Financially it represented a true jump in the dark. Signing up for my new position cost me a 50 percent cut in my income, and I had to buy my way to a very expensive partnership status. I could not understand how I suddenly became a masochist, enjoying inflicting pain and suffering to myself.

I had complete faith and trust in my ability to overcome the difficulty of the situation and to establish my new career. The driving force behind my decision was a deep-seated desire to pursue a new career in the medical field that would allow me to fully express my true aspirations and passions. Cape Cod offered the opportunity for me to fulfill my passion and my preferences in the field of gynecology but also forced me to discover and express other skills and qualities that are well above and beyond my medical ones while motivating me to write this book.

During these intense twenty-three years on Cape Cod, I have learned many painful lessons. As a result, I became a more mature person and professional figure, adding layers of knowledge and appreciation for who I am and my ability to move forward in life. The outcome entailed a profound personal and professional transformation, characterized by deepened wisdom and an enhanced self-awareness, accentuating my capacity to navigate the complexities of life with utmost competence and growth.

I love the change and the transformation that I have endured in the process. I feel like the phoenix, rising from my own ashes. I died right here to resurrect into a different person, emotionally stronger and a more well-rounded professional—not just a physician, but a true healer.

In this very moment, I shed my former self and embraced the profound journey of resurrection. I emerge anew—a person imbued with emotional strength, a beacon of compassion, and a masterful healer.

Beyond the confines of my role as a physician, I transcend the boundaries of conventional practice to embody the essence of true healing. With a soul ablaze and a mind honed by diverse knowledge, I embark on a path that encompasses the holistic well-being of those entrusted to my care. I shall be the catalyst of profound transformations, mending not only physical wounds but also the depths of the human spirit. In this rebirth, I forge a destiny as a well-rounded professional guardian of health, a champion of empathy, and a bearer of healing wisdom.

SECTION I

MY PERSONAL AND PROFESSIONAL EXPERIENCE WITH HPV

CHAPTER ONE

THE JOURNEY OF THE PHOENIX

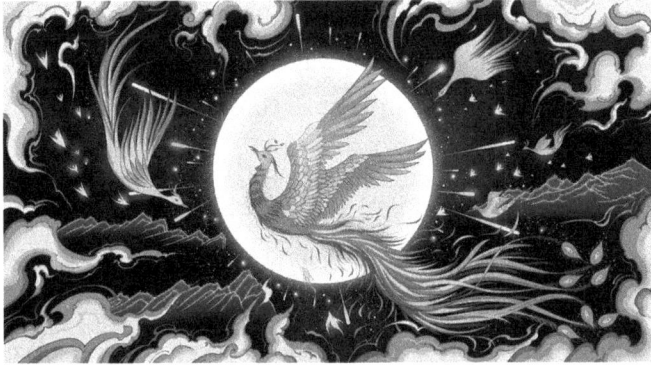

While working on Cape Cod presented many complexities, an additional event significantly impacted my personal life. In November 2011, twenty-two years into my marriage, I had a traumatic experience that shook my level of confidence right to its roots.

The move from Tennessee to the Cape had represented a radical change in my family life and relationship with my husband. That shift was exacerbated when I learned the truth about him conducting a *second life*. I received in the mail unconfutable evidence of his wrongdoing. My husband immediately became estranged—an alienated person pretending to be a good husband and a family man. He delivered one lie after another. It was an escalating process of betrayal that I had to end immediately.

My home, my business, everything I had worked so hard for was in jeopardy. I had to face the new painful reality indicating that my marriage was over. We were done! The divorce was final just ten months later.

Looking back at the last ten years, I realized the extent of the emotional neglect and psychological abuse that I sustained through the relationship. I felt like I had been taking a daily amount of poison small enough not to be noticed, but deadly in the end. I was isolated from the rest of my original family, living so far away from home in another country. I was manipulated and forced into silence by my husband's subtle but effective demeaning behavior. And if this was not bad enough, for eight long years I was denied any chance for intimacy. He was always able to find an excuse to discourage me from getting closer.

The feeling of being rejected and the refusal of any physical contact by the man who I was so completely in love with felt so hurtful and wrong. The pain and emotional distress caused by this situation was abyssal. I felt I was not worthy of his love and attention anymore. My experience left a bitter and sour taste in my mouth just like swallowing my own bile.

It kept on happening. I finally quit trying. I lost hope. I could not accept the thought that he was not in love with me anymore. I could not accept the idea that the love we exchanged for so many years vanished.

Who was this man lying next to me?

My dream of everlasting love was lost forever. I had not done anything wrong. I did not deserve this. I was not in a happy place, and I could not endure this situation any longer. I had too much love and respect for myself to be able to tolerate it.

Finally, the wind of change, transformation, and renewal started blowing again for me.

Two years after my divorce was final, my healing process kicked into a higher gear. My emotional, mental, and physical body reached a new level of balance and well-being together with my heightened level of confidence. I felt strong enough to spread my wings, experiencing total freedom and optimism for the new life I was about to embark on.

I had to learn how to trust another man, and that was the most difficult block to remove. I realized that I had to open my heart first to find a new companion. Once the process was complete, my new relationship took place.

Peter was charming and funny, handsome, and intriguing enough to make me feel like I wanted to know him more. I felt young and vibrant again, ready for a fresh start. I was introduced to his beautiful family and siblings. I got really close to his mom with whom I shared a deep love and sense of appreciation. It was with great anticipation mixed with a strong feeling of insecurity that I terminated my very long, ten-year period of complete abstinence from sexual activity.

I felt vulnerable and excited with the prospect of sharing my love and intimacy with my new partner. Peter was kind and understanding. He never made me feel pressed or threatened. We both eased into the new reality of our relationship with joy and a great sense of respect and complicity.

The world was a beautiful place to explore again with courage and determination. It was fun to be together, and we started craving each other's time and attention. We met regularly, and he introduced me to his kids. We felt like family.

There was excitement, and we both invested a lot of time and energy into strengthening our relationship. His passion for me was strong, and he always tried his best to help me achieve a complete state of ecstasy. I was truly pleased with his genuine interest and the level of affection that he showed me. Our relationship was intense for the first nine months, but it was not an easy path for me.

I slowly realized that we were not heading in the right direction. I never felt I was a real part of his life or world. After the initial months when he was present and attentive, the situation took the wrong turn. I was neglected again. I often felt like I was an accessory, a beautiful object that he would occasionally pull from the shelf and dust off. I was not involved in any of his decisions; there was no planning for the future—only living day by day. I felt I was not part of his plan.

I was hitting a wall again. The negative experience with him had the effect of renewing old wounds, causing a great level of disappointment mixed with despair.

I spent days thinking about what to do, trying to decide.

I was able to go into the deepest part of myself to see how I really felt about this relationship. I had to face the truth devoid of expectations and illusions. At the end of my intimate journey, I came to realize this was not the relationship I wanted. He was not the right person for me.

I had tried hard enough to convey my disappointment to him, to explain my reasons, giving him the opportunity to change. I quickly learned he was not receptive to the change. I called him on the phone just before Christmas to announce my decision to end our relationship. I spent my entire night crying, feeling so bad about myself but firmly convinced I had made the right choice. I had to stop the pain.

He was not comfortable with my decision, and he was determined to conquer my heart again.

He asked me to have one more date.

We sat down at a restaurant, and that evening he asked me to marry him.

I declined.

CHAPTER TWO

ON THE CAPE COD CANAL

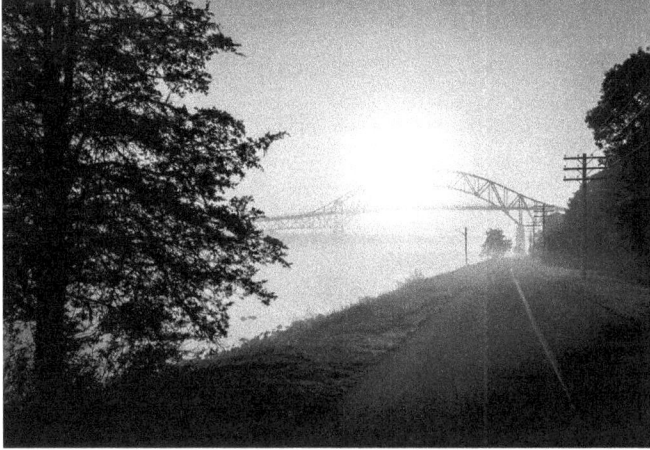

I never resumed a loving relationship with Peter, but we remained good friends for some time after.

We met again in the spring, just a few months after our previous meeting. The sun was gently warming the air, casting a golden hue over everything it touched. The sound of the water rushing through the canal created a soothing backdrop, as if nature itself was orchestrating a calming symphony. The trees were beginning to bloom, their delicate blossoms adding splashes of color to the scene.

As we sat on the bench, a comfortable silence settled between us, carrying the weight of unspoken memories and the joy of reconnecting. The world around us seemed to fade away, leaving only the two of us lost in the moment.

Peter appeared to be very quiet. Looking at me with a serious expression on his face, he announced he had been diagnosed with an advanced stage of cancer of his tongue. One day he realized he was having a really hard time swallowing and felt something was seriously wrong. He saw a specialist who diagnosed a large mass on the back of his tongue, obstructing his pharynx. A biopsy revealed the mass was malignant, and it was caused by the presence of a high-risk strain of HPV, specifically HPV 16, the leading cause of this type of cancer.

"I need to start a long treatment with chemotherapy and radiation," Peter stated. "The cancer could take a toll on my life if I don't start the treatment right away."

I felt chills going down my spine. I went blank for a moment, unable to speak and in a state of shock. My heart sank as I absorbed his words. The tranquility of the spring day suddenly felt shattered, and a heavy cloud of sadness enveloped us. His quiet demeanor and serious expression painted a stark contrast to the peaceful surroundings we were in.

I searched for the right words, my mind racing to find a way to offer comfort and support in the face of such devastating news. The weight of the diagnosis hung in the air, a reminder of life's fragility and the unpredictable nature of our journeys.

"I'm so sorry to hear that," I finally managed to say, my voice carrying a mixture of empathy and concern. "I can't even begin to imagine what you're going through."

Peter nodded slowly, his eyes reflecting a mix of emotions: fear, uncertainty, and perhaps even a hint of acceptance. He began to share the details of his diagnosis, explaining the treatment options being considered and the challenges ahead.

I listened attentively, offering a sympathetic ear as he opened up about his fears and hopes. The canal's turbulent water seemed to mirror the tumultuous emotions swirling within us. Despite the gravity of the situation, our connection remained strong, a testament to the depth of our friendship.

As the sun continued its descent, casting long shadows that seemed to mirror the uncertainty of the future, we talked about the importance of seeking support, both from medical professionals and from friends and family. I assured him he wouldn't be facing this battle alone—I would be there every step of the way, as would others who cared about him.

I was expecting to hear from him soon, but a few weeks passed before I got a call.

We met again along the bank of the Cape Cod Canal.

The salty breeze carried a sense of nostalgia as we stood next to the water. The air was crisp, and the sound of seagulls echoed in the distance. The canal's tranquil waters stretched out before us, reflecting the sky's ever-changing hues. The familiar feeling of reconnection warmed our hearts.

As we walked along the bank, the rhythmic clapping of the water against the shore provided a soothing backdrop to our conversation. The serene beauty and expansive views of the canal offered the perfect setting for reflection and contemplation.

He looked thinner and older; he was going through extensive medical treatment. Peter had to stop working and was unable to drive; the chemo was causing extreme nausea and constant vomiting. He felt exhausted all the time. I could see the toll his condition had taken. His movements were slower, and there was a vulnerability in his eyes that hadn't been there before.

Unable to eat, Peter underwent a procedure in which a feeding tube was placed at the level of his stomach to allow for some nourishment. It served as a lifeline, a connection to nourishment and sustenance that his body needed. It was a tangible representation of his resilience, the determination to find a way forward despite the obstacles that life had thrown his way.

The weight of his recent surgical procedure was evident, and it was a stark reminder of the challenges he was facing. His life was totally devastated and turned upside down.

We met again one more time at the end of his treatment. He made a full recovery, although he looked much older. There was some gravity in his voice that was totally new to me. It felt like it was coming from a remote place. His perspective on life, as well as his emotional world, were seriously shaken. I noticed a richer level of maturity, which made him look even more interesting, more intriguing than ever before.

During the entire length of our meeting, he kept his eyes down. His face had a sad expression and his words sounded heavy when he said: "Lucia, I am ashamed to tell you I have been sharing my bed with another woman. She has been the one who has been helping me with transportation to the hospital and back through the entire length of my illness. I am not in love with her, and I have been waiting for the right moment to tell her the truth. I need to be totally honest with you, and I want you to know about my new reality."

The weight of his words hung heavily in the air as he finally looked up, his sad expression meeting my gaze. The atmosphere around us seemed to shift, as if the weight of his confession had altered the very energy of the space we occupied.

I felt a mixture of surprise and confusion along with a tinge of sadness at his admission. The gravity of the situation was palpable, and his voice carried a sense of remorse and regret as he spoke those difficult words. It was clear he was struggling to find the right way to express his feelings and explain his actions.

His vulnerability was evident, and honesty in his admission was both painful and admirable. I could see the internal struggle Peter was facing, the conflict between the desire to be truthful and the fear of the consequences of his actions. It was a raw and unfiltered moment where his true emotions were laid bare before me. I could certainly understand where he was coming from.

It was only a few weeks earlier when he asked me to marry him; how could he forget about his feelings so quickly?

He kept in touch with me over the phone a few times to let me know he was trying hard to end the relationship with his caregiver. Weeks went by, and his situation remained unchanged. He was totally entangled and unable to end his one-sided love affair. Waiting for him to free himself from a relationship in which he was not in love was emotionally draining and challenging for me. My weariness stemmed from a place of concern and care for his well-being.

It was difficult to witness someone I cared about in a situation that did not bring him happiness or align with his true feelings. I felt my own emotions and needs were valid, and it was important to prioritize my own well-being while also supporting him in his journey. I made a significant choice to place myself as a priority by reserving the right to explore new relationships, and I communicated this decision openly to him. This marked a crucial milestone in my journey toward self-care, demonstrating my commitment to pursuing the happiness and fulfillment I truly deserved.

Regrettably, he did not provide the supportive response I had hoped for. Instead, he chose to disengage completely. His lack of communication thereafter indicated a clear conclusion to our relationship. Without any subsequent contact or calls, it became evident that our connection had come to an end.

Living this experience, even indirectly through my partner, had the effect of opening my mind to the reality of thousands of men and women whose lives are totally devastated by the presence of an HPV-related cancer.

I started wondering why so few people are aware of the existence of the HPV virus and the risks derived from harboring the virus in their system. Through this painful personal and emotional experience, I learned how important it is to always consider the potential danger of contracting a sexually transmitted disease through a new relationship.

I felt so vulnerable knowing I could have been exposed to this potentially serious illness, and I realized how lucky I was when I made the decision prior to dating again to give myself the HPV vaccine to prevent a possible infection with it through a new partner. I am so grateful for the fact I was aware of the risk of contracting HPV and for taking the necessary steps to prevent the infection.

In my medical career and during the past few decades, I have seen a growing number of patients struggling with the diagnosis of HPV. HPV has a stigma because it is considered a sexually transmitted disease. I was able to witness, through my partner's life experience at that time, how insidious and devastating it can be to develop cancer related to it.

In my many-decades-long practice of gynecology, I have encountered hundreds of patients of any age and social extraction whose lives have been affected directly or indirectly through their partner by the presence of HPV-related conditions.

I made my decision to write this book to increase awareness around the issue of HPV infection as well as the real potential risks. I cannot stress enough the importance for men and women of any age to consider the HPV vaccine as a primary as well as a secondary preventive measure. It is my intention to launch a campaign that will allow patients full access to the HPV vaccine independently from age, sex, and social status.

SECTION II

HOW HPV CAN AFFECT THE HUMAN BODY: HEALTH CONCERNS AND TREATMENT OPTIONS

CHAPTER THREE

OVERVIEW OF HIGH-RISK HPV

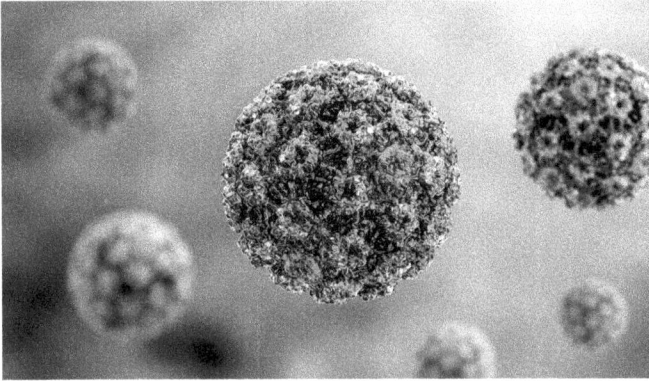

HUMAN PAPILLOMAVIRUS AMONG US: WHAT IS IT?

Human papillomavirus (HPV) is primarily transmitted through sexual contact, including vaginal, anal, and oral sex. When an individual engages in sexual activity with an infected partner, the virus can be transmitted and establish an infection in the host's genital area. The virus can also be transmitted through intimate skin-to-skin contact without sexual intercourse. HPV is highly contagious and can be passed on silently. There are, in fact, no noticeable symptoms or evident skin lesions in the early stages.

Almost 80 million Americans are infected with HPV, the most common viral STD in the world (Van Dyne, et al. 2018). Anyone who is sexually active can be at risk for HPV, regardless of their marital status, age, or social and economic conditions. HPV is highly prevalent, and most sexually active individuals will encounter the virus at some point in their lives.

The virus can be present in the body in a dormant state, meaning that it has infected the cells but is not actively reproducing. The malignant potential of the virus is due to its ability to multiply and spread in the affected tissue, causing the disease.

It is unpredictable to know when it will become active.

Many people can clear the infection on their own without experiencing any health problems; however, it can take up to two years for the patient to develop immunity to the virus. (Moscicki, et al. 1998).

According to the CDC: "Each year in the United States, about 47,984 new cases of cancer are found in parts of the body where human papillomavirus (HPV) is often found: 26,280 among females, and 21,704 among males. HPV causes about 37,800 of these cancers. Cervical cancer is the most common HPV-associated cancer among women, and oropharyngeal cancers (cancers of the back of the throat, including the base of the tongue and tonsils) are the most common among men."[1] (https://www.cdc.gov/cancer/hpv/cases.html)

Women reporting a new sex partner are at increased risk of contracting an infection with the virus, affecting any age (Proma, et al. 2021). It is reported that 80 percent of women will acquire HPV by age fifty.[2] (Braaten and Laufer, 2008).

It's important to note that HPV can also be transmitted through skin-to-skin contact, so sexual intercourse is not the only mode of transmission. The virus can be transmitted through other means, such as from mother to child during childbirth.

Given the potential for HPV to lead to cervical and other reproductive tract cancers, vaccination against HPV is an essential preventive measure, especially for individuals before they become sexually active.

Regular screening, such as Pap smears and HPV testing, is also of vital importance for early detection and timely intervention in high-risk populations, including sexually active individuals and those with a history of HPV infection.

The Link Between HPV and Certain Cancers

HPV can remain dormant in the body for as long as thirty-five years, escaping recognition from the immune system. Typically, any time the immune response is suppressed in the body, it can cause the activation of the HPV malignant potential. When it becomes active, it will start making copies of itself by changing the DNA programming of the host cell.

The ability of the virus to penetrate the nucleus of the cell, changing the DNA, makes this virus harmful because that is how the risk of cancer increases exponentially. High-risk types of HPV are associated with an increased risk of certain cancers. Low-risk strains are more likely to cause benign conditions, such as genital warts.

High-risk HPV is a DNA virus of high *oncogenic potential*, which means that it can cause cancer if not monitored carefully. There are 228 different types of HPV.

Each type of HPV is assigned a number for identification.

There are 15 different types of HPV that fit the high-risk category: 16, 18, 31, 33, 35, 39, 45, 51, 52, 56, 58, 59, 68, 73, and 82.

HPV 16 and 18 account for 70 percent of cases of cervical cancer.[3] (James Radosevich, Ph.D. "HPV and cancer" Springer, 2012)

Besides cervical cancer, high-risk HPV has also been associated with other types of cancer, including:

- Anal cancer – HPV is a significant risk factor for anal cancer, especially in men who have sex with men.

- Oropharyngeal (mouth and throat) cancer – HPV infection, particularly with certain high-risk types like HPV-16, is a known risk factor for cancers of the mouth and throat.

- Vulvar and vaginal cancer – High-risk HPV can also contribute to the development of vulvar and vaginal cancers in women.

- Penile cancer – In men, high-risk HPV infection can increase the risk of developing penile cancer.

It's essential to note that while high-risk HPV increases the risk of these cancers, it does not necessarily mean that an infected individual will develop cancer. The body's immune response plays a crucial role in clearing the infection in many cases. Regular screenings, early detection, and appropriate medical interventions can help prevent or treat HPV-related cancers effectively.

Vaccination, such as with the HPV vaccine Gardasil, against high-risk HPV types has proven to be a valuable preventive measure in reducing the incidence of HPV-associated cancers. According to the CDC: "The HPV vaccine works extremely well. In the 10 years after the vaccine was recommended in 2006 in the United States, quadrivalent type HPV infections decreased by 86% in female teens aged 14 to 19 years and 71% in women in their early 20s. Research has also shown that fewer teens and young adults are getting genital warts and that cervical precancers are decreasing since HPV vaccines have been in use in the United States. A decrease in vaccine-type prevalence, genital warts, and cervical precancers have also been observed in other countries with HPV vaccination programs."[4] (https://www.cdc.gov/vaccines/vpd/hpv/hcp/safety-effectiveness.html)

HPV AND OTHER COMMON INFECTIONS OF THE REPRODUCTIVE TRACT

The association between some bacteria and the subsequent production of cancer is well known for bacteria like *Helicobacter pylori*, or H. pylori, a common source of stomach ulcers, cancer, and gastritis. H. pylori overgrowth in our body can also increase the risk of non-Hodgkin's lymphoma in humans.

The more-than-one-hundred species of the bacteria *Streptococcus* (Strep) can release factors and chemical mediators that have the effect of weakening the integrity of tissues, allowing for an easier penetration of the virus. This is true at the level of the oral cavity as well as the vaginal tissue.

Strep and HPV are the best of allies, promoting significant structural changes with the effect of facilitating cancer development and progression. Strep has been associated with the presence of several epithelial cancers of the lung, breast, colon, and prostate.

Some strains of Streptococcus and *Staphylococcus* bacteria, which can be present in our digestive tract and the vaginal canal, have been associated with an increased risk of adenocarcinoma of the colon.

A folate-deficient diet together with an increased intake of sugar can stimulate the Strep present in the mouth to release the dangerous chemical *acetaldehyde*, as can smoking and alcohol consumption. Acetaldehyde is produced and released by bacteria and can damage the DNA inside human cells, thereby increasing the risk of cancers.

According to the National Library of Medicine: "Bacterial vaginosis is the most prevalent vaginitis in females of reproductive age, with an estimated occurrence ranging from 5% to 70%."[5] (https://medlineplus.gov/vaginitis.html).

"The prevalence of bacterial vaginosis among females fluctuates from 20% to 60% across various countries."[6] (https://www.ncbi.nlm.nih.gov/books/NBK459216).

Bacterial vaginosis (BV) is not exactly considered a true infection, but a condition in which there is a shift from benign to more harmful bacteria colonizing the genital tract.

Poly-Microbial Interaction With HPV

The presence of a concomitant bacterial infection of the vagina might facilitate an infection with HPV. HPV 51 and 52 are often associated with bacterial vaginosis.[7] (Dahoud, et al. 2019).

The exposure to smoking or alcohol will not only cause more damage to the tissue, but also produce cancer-inducing bio-products, such as the above-mentioned acetaldehyde and other chemicals that suppress the immune system function. Additionally, drinking alcohol and smoking can cause direct damage to the host DNA, increasing the chance for mutations of the genetic material that could lead to the onset of cancer.

Chlamydia, which can be sexually transmitted, has been associated with adenocarcinoma of the lungs as well as an increased risk of lymphoma.

To end this chapter on a good note, it is interesting to know the intake of coffee could offer some protection against Oropharyngeal cancer, as shown by a systematic review and metanalysis published by the National Library of Medicine in 2017.[8] (https://pmc.ncbi.nlm.nih.gov/articles/PMC5694177)

HPV Diagnosis: Understanding Limitations and Best Practices

The diagnosis of Human Papillomavirus (HPV) currently relies on tests available exclusively for women, typically performed during a Pap smear. Unfortunately, there are no FDA-approved HPV tests for men currently. Additionally, existing HPV tests can only detect fourteen high-risk HPV types, meaning a negative result does not exclude the possibility of infection with other high-risk HPV types not identified by these tests.[9] (https://pmc.ncbi.nlm.nih.gov/articles/PMC3889747.)

Dormant HPV Infections

It's essential to understand that HPV tests may not detect the virus if it is in a dormant state, where it is not actively replicating or proliferating within the tissue. This limitation highlights the importance of regular monitoring, even with negative test results.

Limitations of Pap Smears

The Pap smear, though a critical diagnostic tool, is not 100 percent accurate and carries the risk of false-negative results. A false negative can occur when an abnormality in cervical or vaginal tissue is present but goes undetected. This is particularly concerning when a Pap smear report indicates a "non-satisfactory" result.

A non-satisfactory Pap smear typically means the sample lacks adequate cells from either the outer cervix or the endocervical canal, making it unrepresentative of the true condition of cervical tissue. This situation is more common in older women, where menopause and aging may cause anatomical changes, such as narrowing of the cervical canal making sampling more challenging. These factors can prevent the detection of abnormal or high-risk cells deeply located inside the cervical canal.

The Need for Annual Exams

In cases where a Pap smear is non-satisfactory or inconclusive, it remains possible for a patient to harbor high-risk HPV types undetected by current tests. Therefore, annual pelvic exams and Pap smears are recommended to monitor any potential changes over time. Regular examinations can help identify subtle or unexpected abnormalities before they progress.

The Role of the Pelvic Exam

A thorough pelvic exam conducted annually is invaluable. During the exam, a healthcare provider carefully inspects the vulva, vaginal canal, and cervix for signs of cancer or pre-cancerous lesions. This comprehensive evaluation also helps detect other abnormalities, including:

- **Uterine, ovarian, and fallopian tube irregularities**

- **Pelvic masses such as tumors, fibroids, or cysts**

- **Pelvic infections**

Additionally, pelvic exams provide an opportunity to identify skin-related conditions such as melanomas, cancer or abnormal pigmentation on the vulva—areas often overlooked by dermatologists.

The Importance of Expertise

The accuracy and reliability of HPV diagnostics heavily depend on the skill and experience of the provider performing the Pap smear and pelvic exam. A well-trained gynecologist plays an irreplaceable role in early detection and preventive care, ensuring abnormalities are identified promptly.

Best Practices for HPV Screening

Given the limitations of current diagnostic tests and the widespread prevalence of HPV, the best approach is to maintain a consistent schedule of annual exams and Pap smears. Regular monitoring allows healthcare providers to catch early changes and take preventive measures before the virus potentially becomes active or leads to complications.

The Disservice to Elder Women

It is imperative that women receive their gynecological exam every year without being discriminated against according to age, insurance coverage, or social status. According to the CDC, the cumulative rate of HPV-related cancers diagnosed in female patients during the years 2017–2021 is higher than 26 out of 100,000 for women aged sixty–sixty-nine.[10] (https://www.cdc.gov/cancer/hpv/diagnosis-by-age.html)

Because of this high rate, I believe it is of utmost importance for older women to continue their surveillance against cancer of the reproductive tract, anus, and oropharynx.

The pelvic exam should be done starting at the time of sexual activity and continue well into older age.

Patients over seventy are often advised that cancer screenings are no longer necessary, which can unintentionally discourage them from attending regular gynecological exams. This can create the misleading perception that age itself offers protection against cancer and other serious conditions, or that treatment options may not be effective or worthwhile in later years.

However, as life expectancy continues to rise, so does the potential for cervical cancer and other HPV-related cancer among women over sixty-five. The Centers for Disease Control and Prevention highlights this concern, noting that women remain at significant risk of cervical cancer until the age of eighty.

Prioritizing routine screenings and preventive care for older women is essential for their health and well-being.

A CDC study highlights that cervical cancer tends to be diagnosed at younger ages than other HPV-associated cancers. The median ages of diagnosis vary by cancer type and gender, with cervical cancer being diagnosed at a median age of fifty. Other median ages include:

- Vaginal and vulvar cancers: sixty-eight years

- Penile cancer: sixty-nine years

- Anal cancer: sixty-four for females, sixty-two for males

- Oropharyngeal cancers: sixty-four for females, sixty-three for males

The study also used cancer registry data to estimate HPV's role in different cancer types, suggesting that HPV is likely responsible for about 91 percent of cervical cancers, 75 percent of vaginal cancers, 69 percent of vulvar cancers, 63 percent of penile cancers, 91 percent of anal cancers, and 70 percent of oropharyngeal cancers. These findings underscore the importance of early and regular screening for HPV-associated cancers across age groups.[11] (https://www.cdc.gov/cancer/hpv/diagnosis-by-age.html)

WHEN THE TEST RESULT IS POSITIVE

The latent state of HPV means that it remains in the body without showing any signs or causing any symptoms.

Individuals may carry the virus unknowingly for a prolonged time, even if they have not been sexually active for a long time.

We need to understand, despite the absence of symptoms, the virus has the potential to become active at some future point.

In my daily gynecological practice, I frequently see patients in their seventies and eighties, many widowed and not sexually active for years yet still testing positive for HPV.

This phenomenon might seem surprising at first glance, but it underscores the unique nature of the HPV virus. Unlike many other infections, HPV can remain dormant and undetectable in the body for decades.

During this latent phase, the virus lies inactive, only to resurface under certain conditions, such as changes in the immune system. This ability of HPV to persist silently for extended periods highlights the importance of regular screenings and awareness, regardless of age or recent sexual activity.

As a medical practitioner, it is crucial to remain vigilant and to inform patients about the possibility of latent HPV and the importance of regular screening and checkups, even in the absence of recent sexual activity. This is especially true for those who test positive for HPV, or who have a history of it, to ensure comprehensive care and reduce the impact of cervical cancer and other HPV-related diseases.

Regular screening and vigilant monitoring are essential for the early detection and timely management of HPV-related complications. Healthcare providers play a crucial role in educating patients about HPV risks and the importance of preventive measures, regardless of their relationship status. By fostering awareness and proactive care, providers can help improve overall reproductive health and significantly reduce the incidence of HPV-associated cancers.

A patient who tests positive for high-risk HPV has an increased likelihood of developing cervical, vaginal, vulvar, anal, or oropharyngeal cancer.

A positive result with HPV in a younger patient population should prompt healthcare providers to consider a complete STI screening because of the heightened risk of having other infections, such as HIV, hepatitis B and C, syphilis, chlamydia, and gonorrhea, which are also considered sexually transmitted conditions.

It is important to recognize that certain sexually transmitted infections (STIs) can alter the environment of the reproductive tract, making it more susceptible to HPV infection. These changes can compromise the natural barriers that protect against viral entry and persistence, increasing the risk of contracting HPV.

This highlights the need for comprehensive sexual health screening and preventive measures, including vaccination and education. By addressing co-existing STIs and promoting preventive strategies, we can take proactive steps to safeguard long-term reproductive and overall health.

As healthcare providers, it is crucial to remain vigilant about the risks associated with HPV and other STIs and to emphasize the importance of regular screening, vaccination, safe sexual practices, and overall sexual health education to reduce the incidence and impact of these infections on individuals and communities.

It is important to offer a program of comprehensive sexual education for teens in school.

Having a positive HPV status indeed places the patient in a different risk category, and this information is crucial for determining appropriate follow-up and management strategies. Depending on the specific HPV type detected and other risk factors, healthcare providers can recommend more frequent screenings, colposcopies, or other preventive measures.

CHAPTER FOUR

HPV-RELATED CANCERS

High-risk HPV types are strongly associated with the development of cervical cancer. Persistent infection with these high-risk types can lead to the gradual transformation of normal cervical cells into precancerous cells and eventually into invasive cervical cancer.

CERVICAL CANCER

Despite the advances in the medical field in terms of the ability to diagnose and treat HPV infection, the rate of cervical cancer is increasing worldwide.

Each year in the U.S., it is estimated that nearly 11,000 women develop cervical cancer (CDC 2023). HPV 16 probably accounts for almost 12 percent of all cancers in women, and cervical cancer represents the second most frequent gynecological malignancy in the world among women of reproductive age.

According to the *Human Papillomavirus and Related Cancers, Summary Report 2010*, among women across the world who are diagnosed with cervical cancer, 52 percent die of that cancer.[12] (https://screening.iarc.fr/atlasHPV.php)

The five-year overall survival rate is 72 percent in North America.

The prognosis of cervical cancer depends on the staging of the tumor. With early detection and treatment, 80–90 percent of women with Stage I cancer and 50–65 percent of women with Stage II cancer are alive five years after the diagnosis.[13] (HPV and cancer, J Radosevich Ph.D., Springer 2019 edition).

"HPV infection has reached a considerable proportion worldwide, particularly among women, in whom it is the primary cause of cancer."[13] (https://pmc.ncbi.nlm.nih.gov/articles/PMC7855977/#B10)   Thus, making HPV a current public health priority.

"With an estimated 291 million HPV-positive women worldwide in 2007, HPV infection has remained one of the most common viral infections in the world."[14] (https://pmc.ncbi.nlm.nih.gov/articles/PMC7855977/#B11)

Screening reduces the mortality rate by more than 50 percent.[15] (https://www.sciencedirect.com/science/article/pii/0091743589900017)

(HPV and Cervical Cancer: Updates on an Established Relationship: Postgraduate Medicine: Vol 120, No 4)[16]

The result of the 2012 U.S. Preventive Services Task Force recommendation that lengthened the screening intervals up to five years in between exams has caused a decrease in the rate of screening for HPV in women ages twenty-one to twenty-nine. According to cancer incidence data from the cancer registry, the rate of cervical cancer has increased up to 11.60 percent from 2012 to 2019 in women ages thirty-five to fifty-four. The most significant increase is seen in women thirty to thirty-four, especially in Hispanic women.

The rate of cervical cancer increases because of women not being screened at an earlier age. The consequent decline in the screening participation of these women, as recommended by their medical provider, has led to an increase of 2.5 percent per year in the rate of cervical cancer. This is quite a disservice, affecting young and vital patients who deserve better care.

Pre-Cancerous Lesions of the Genital Tract

The process of interaction of HPV with the DNA of the host cells has the effect of changing their look on the Pap smear. There are three distinct levels of precancerous lesions of the cervix: mild, moderate, and severe.

Older women have the tendency to harbor the virus in their system longer than younger women, who will instead clear the infection more easily. Statistics show that 25 percent of mild pre-cancerous lesions will convert to normal. The other 25 percent of cases will get worse over time. The remaining 50 percent will stay the same.

Dysplasia is a condition that can develop not only at the level of the cervix but also in the vaginal tissue as well as in the vulva. There are different grades of precancerous lesions of the cervix called *Dysplasia*: mild, moderate, and severe dysplasia.

Mild Dysplasia

A mild precancerous lesion is called *mild dysplasia* or CIN I. At this stage, the cells look abnormal, but they are still organized in a regular pattern that is close to normal. The nucleus inside the cell becomes larger than usual, revealing an increased activity at the transcriptional level.

A mild dysplasia is managed with observation because of the tendency of the abnormality to resolve on its own, especially in younger women. The probability of regression with Low-grade Squamous Intraepithelial Lesion (LSIL), also called *mild dysplasia*, is 61 percent at twelve months and 91 percent at thirty-six months.

Moderate dysplasia represents a more advanced pre-cancerous lesion affecting the genital tract, including the cervical, vaginal, and vulvar tissues. These lesions are less likely to regress spontaneously and typically require surgical excision to prevent progression.

Severe dysplasia, on the other hand, involves cellular changes that closely resemble cancerous cells. However, unlike invasive cancer, these lesions tend to remain localized and lack the ability to spread to the lymphatic system. This makes them amenable to complete removal through surgical intervention.

It's important to note that as the degree of cellular abnormality increases, so is the likelihood of the lesion progressing to invasive cancer. Early detection and timely treatment are therefore critical in preventing the development of cancer and ensuring better health outcomes.

Once the positive HPV status has been detected in a Pap smear, the patient is evaluated with a further study called *colposcopy*—a procedure in which the provider examines the cervix, vaginal walls, and vulva with an instrument called a *colposcope*, designed to magnify the view of the cervix and further into the vagina. Using the colposcope, a microscopic view of the genital tract aids in the detection of fine abnormality of the tissue that is otherwise not detectable with normal sight.

In a study of 160 patients, the diagnostic accuracy of the colposcopy was 96.3 percent compared with the 82.2 percent accuracy of a Pap smear alone (Najib, et al. 2020). According to Dr. Joanna Swiderska-Kiec from the Dept. of OB/GYN at the Medical University of Warsaw (Poland), HPV testing combined with colposcopy is the most effective method for detecting CIN lesions (Swiderska-Kiec, et al. 2020).

At the end of the colposcopy of the cervix, vaginal walls, and vulva, the provider typically *biopsies*—obtains a tiny fragment of—the tissue and sends it to the pathology lab to confirm the abnormality and establish a definite diagnosis.

Since the introduction of the colposcopy following the detection of an abnormal cytology, the incidence of cervical cancer in the United

States has decreased substantially in those patients who were treated (Massad, et al. 2013).

Treatment of Precancerous Lesions of the Cervix and Genital Tracts

Cryotherapy

Patients who do not clear the abnormality and who show persistence of the lesion over time are candidates for an elective procedure called *cryotherapy*. During the procedure, the provider destroys the lesion by freezing the superficial layer of tissue where the abnormal cells are located. This procedure is only indicated in women who have had a "satisfactory" colposcopy and a negative endo-cervical specimen.

The procedure is considered very safe and is well tolerated.

LEEP/ Cone Biopsy

This surgery is effective in removing the lesion when "the margins of the surgical specimen are clear" from residual abnormality.

The procedure typically does not go further than two centimeters deep into the cervix.

It does pose a small risk of subsequent complications, such as infertility due to scarring of the cervical canal or *incompetent cervix*, which could lead to pregnancy loss, most commonly around sixteen weeks of estimated gestational age.

Another option, mainly in women who are past reproduction, is to remove the uterus altogether through a hysterectomy to minimize the risk of cervical cancer in the future. Women need to know, even after hysterectomy, surveillance against the virus must remain high due to the possibility of a recurrence of the viral activity in the future, with a possible new onset of a lesion at the level of either the vaginal walls or vulva.

It is not unusual for the patient to develop vaginal cancer after hysterectomy that was done for a precancerous lesion of the cervix due to HPV.

This was the case for one of my patients.

She was in fact diagnosed with an aggressive stage of vaginal cancer due to HPV just six months after she had undergone a total hysterectomy to treat a precancerous lesion of her cervix. The cancer was invasive and required additional therapy with radiation.

Statistics show that 65 percent of women who had a hysterectomy for a precancerous lesion of the cervix are subsequently diagnosed with a precancerous lesion in their vagina.

The use of vaginal estrogen therapy has been associated with a high rate of resolution, up to 90 percent, and it is not associated with the high-grade toxicity of other chemical treatments, including one known as 5FU (Rossi, 2018).

Lichen Sclerosis

Lichen sclerosis (LS) is a common chronic inflammatory skin condition that can affect various parts of the body, including the vulva. It is more commonly seen in postmenopausal women, but it can also occur in premenopausal women, men, and children.

Symptoms of lichen sclerosis in the vulva may include:

- *Itching*: Itching is the most common symptom and can range from mild to severe, leading to significant discomfort.

- *White patches*: The affected skin may appear white, shiny, and thin. The skin may also become fragile and easily injured.

- *Pain or soreness*: Some women may experience pain or soreness, especially during sexual intercourse or while urinating.

- *Bleeding or tearing*: Due to the thinning and fragility of the affected skin, there may be occasional bleeding or tearing of the tissue.

- *Scarring*: Over time, the inflammation and damage caused by lichen sclerosis can lead to scarring and deformity of the labia with agglutination and narrowing of the vaginal opening that will eventually interfere with sexual functioning.

In extreme cases when the scarring of the skin is left untreated, there will be a significant obstruction to the flow of urine in these patients, requiring a surgical release.

The skin condition is much worse in postmenopausal women due to the lack of estrogen in their system, which produces a decrease in collagen and elastin production as well as a decrease in the blood supply to the tissue of the vulva and the vagina. Both organs will experience a significant amount of thinning as well as a loss of moisture because of the hormonal deprivation.

The exact cause of lichen sclerosis is not fully understood, but it is believed to be related to an autoimmune process. It is not contagious and cannot be transmitted through sexual contact. There is some clinical evidence to suggest an association between lichen sclerosis and HPV.

A study published by the *International Journal of Dermatology* in February 2017 showed an 8 percent association between HPV and lichen sclerosis with HPV 16 being the most prevalent strain involved.[17] (https://onlinelibrary.wiley.com/doi/10.1111/ijd.13697)

In these women, the Pap smear might not be able to show a positive high-risk HPV status, and the positivity for the virus will show only on the tissue biopsy done to confirm the diagnosis of a lichen.

The provider needs to be aware of the possible involvement of the HPV virus in the diagnosis of HPV. They must ask specifically for the pathologist to submit the tissue provided with the biopsy to test for the presence of the HPV virus.

Women need to be aware of the possibility of developing cancer at the level of their vulva; therefore, it is important to check the area very carefully at least two to three times yearly. Any change in the color, texture of the skin, or pigmentation; any growth of tissue; and any symptom of pain, irritation, or itching should be reported to the medical provider.

I will never forget Mary, a forty-year-old patient who presented to my office for her initial visit with me because she discovered a growth of tissue on her vulva. She had listened to a radio program that recommended women check their vulvas for any suspicious lesions.

She followed the advice and, sure enough, she found a spot she never knew was there before. She decided to make an appointment to see me in my office. I performed a biopsy, and it revealed she had cancer of the vulva. Fortunately, it was caught it at an early stage. Surgery cured her condition.

Another patient came to my office complaining of some spotting she believed was coming from her urinary tract. She had undergone a hysterectomy many years ago for a precancerous lesion of her cervix due to HPV. Upon examination, she was diagnosed with an ulcerated, advanced-stage melanoma of the vulva, she has experienced several recurrences of her cancer and she continues to undergo medical treatment for it.

OTHER CANCERS INDUCED BY HIGH-RISK HPV

High-risk HPV can also be responsible for other kinds of cancer. The two most common cancers are oropharyngeal and anal.

Oropharyngeal cancer

Oropharyngeal cancer refers to cancer that develops in the oropharynx, which includes the back of the throat, the base of the tongue, and the tonsils. HPV infection, particularly with high-risk strains such as HPV 16 and HPV 18, has been strongly linked to the development of oropharyngeal cancer; in fact, it has been implicated in more than 60 percent of U.S. cases. (Fakhry, et al. 2008)

Again, not all individuals exposed to high-risk HPV will develop oropharyngeal cancer. The virus's presence is just one of several factors that can influence the risk of cancer development. Other factors, such as smoking, excessive alcohol consumption, and overall immune system health also play a role.

The most common clinical signs and symptoms that may indicate the presence of cancer are: difficulty swallowing, persistent cough, hoarseness, blood in the sputum, and pain or burning in the mouth.

In the late stage of the disease the lymph nodes in the neck will be swollen as a sign of the lymphatic spread of the tumor (Radosevich, 2019).

"The assessment of SEER research database between 1992–2008 shows that the rate of oropharyngeal cancer in the black male population is higher than in the general population, estimated at 18.67 cases/100.000." (James Radosevich, PH.D "HPV and cancer" Springer edition, July 4, 2019)

The USA National Cancer Institute's Surveillance Epidemiology and End Results (SEER) database also shows that "the age-adjusted incidence of oropharyngeal cancer increased 2–4% annually from 1973 to 2001, particularly among younger adults—more frequently male and Caucasian—and may develop in individuals who do not have a concurrent risk of tobacco or alcohol use." (Radosevich, 2019)

"Risk factors for these patients include younger age of sexual activity and increased numbers of sexual partners"[18] (Souza, et al. 2007, 2010; Gillison, et al. 2008; Heck, et al 2010, Smith, et al. 2004)

According to the CDC, there are 21,474 cancers of the oropharynx diagnosed each year.

The incidence is higher in men, with 17,832 new cases, compared to 3,642 in females.

Around 70 percent of these cancers are directly related to HPV. (https://www.cdc.gov/cancer/hpv/cases.html)

The use of alcohol or smoking can damage our DNA, affecting the ability of the immune system to fight the infection with HPV.

The Streptococcus bacteria commonly present in the mouth can release acetaldehyde (AA) when they meet even a small amount of alcohol, such as that found in mouthwash.

Acetaldehyde is a toxic compound that over time can damage the DNA of the oral cells, increasing the risk of developing cancer.

A diet deficient in folic acid and high in sugar can increase the risk of cancer by stimulating the streptococcus to release AA in the oral mucosa.

Furthermore, the use of immunosuppressant therapy for conditions like ulcerative colitis, psoriasis, and eczema can significantly increase the risk of developing HPV-related cancers in the affected individual.

On a positive note, a pooled analysis of case-control studies supports the hypothesis of an inverse association between caffeinated coffee drinking and OP cancer risk. (https://pmc.ncbi.nlm.nih.gov/articles/ PMC3047460)

This means coffee intake may have a protective effect against cancer of the mouth and throat because of its antioxidant effect.

The study shows "Caffeinated coffee intake was inversely related with the risk of cancer of the oral cavity and pharynx (OP): the ORs were 0.96 (95% CI 0.94–0.98) for an increment of one cup per day and 0.61 (95% CI 0.47–0.80) in drinkers of >4 cups per day vs. non-drinkers."

Head and neck cancers can be cured 90 percent of the time when diagnosed at an early stage.

The five-year prognosis of survival goes down to 50 percent, depending on the stage of the tumor.

The most common treatment recommended is radiation therapy.

The most common side effects reported are dry mouth; hoarseness; difficulty chewing, tasting, and talking; and limited movement of the tongue and jaw.

There is also an increased risk of developing thrush—yeast infection of the mouth— and aseptic necrosis of the jaw, which can lead to fracture.

HPV 16 is the most common type of HPV associated with this kind of cancer in men.

Anal Cancer

Anal cancer makes up about 2 percent of all gastrointestinal cancers, and its incidence has been rising in many western countries—the U.S., parts of Europe, Australia, and South America—though it remains relatively stable in Asian populations.

Current estimates in the United States suggest about 9,760 new cases and 1,870 deaths from anal cancer in 2023.

Overall, women have higher incidence rates than men. Since the late 1990s, the incidence of anal squamous cell carcinoma (ASCC) has increased significantly across all ages, with the fastest growth among individuals aged thirty-five–forty-nine, followed by those fifty–sixty-four, and with older women (greater or more than sixty-five years) experiencing the highest rates.

The primary factor behind these rising numbers appears to be increasing HPV infection rates.[19] (https://pmc.ncbi.nlm.nih.gov/articles/PMC10047250)

HPV is the reason anal cancer incidence is higher in the younger population. The most common symptom is rectal bleeding or a sensation of growth in the anal area. Chemoradiation therapy is the treatment of choice initially.

Around 70 percent of HPV infections heal on their own within one year, and 90 percent heal within two years. (American Cancer Society, 2024). It is recommended to screen the anal area carefully, especially in women who test positive for HPV or who have a history of HPV-related lesions in the genital tract.

CHAPTER FIVE

NATURAL COURSE OF THE HPV-INDUCED DISEASE

We have already established that HPV can remain latent in the body for many years. It is unpredictable when the virus will become active, as several conditions might trigger the replication process. Stress, getting sick, and taking medications such as steroids or other immunosuppressant agents might lower or prevent the immune system from controlling the HPV.

HOW CANCERS DEVELOP

Once active, the virus can move from the deep layers of the affected tissue where it commonly resides to the more superficial ones, where it can be easily detected. The virus initiates a highly efficient and rapid replication cycle characterized by an accelerated rate of proliferation within its host, leading to an increased production of viral particles. This heightened replication activity enables the virus to surface within the infected tissues, making itself more detectable by immune cells and specialized laboratory tests designed to identify its presence.

The active virus stimulates the superficial cells of the tissue involved to exit the resting phase, which is the normal status of these cells. It forces them to proliferate to accommodate the viral needs and requirements. The superficial cells stimulated to grow and multiply by the presence of the active HPV will look abnormal and are called *atypical*. In other words, the virus can transform a normal cell that has reached its maturity and resting cycle into a busy manufacturer, producing and assembling thousands of new viral units every day. The infected cells are enslaved to the high metabolic requirements of the virus.

The infected cells display an astonishing ability to undergo rapid and uncontrolled replication. This relentless pace overwhelms the immune cells, leaving them unable to effectively contain the viral spread. Consequently, the immune response becomes compromised, allowing the virus to escalate its damaging potential unchecked.

The body's defense mechanisms are significantly challenged as they struggle to keep up with the virus's formidable reproduction rate, ultimately leading to increased disease severity and potential complications. The presence of atypical cells in a Pap smear is a red flag, alerting the provider to further test and identify the problem. The cells look dysplastic as an effect of the HPV virus interacting with the genetic material in the cells, causing significant damage as well as inducing chromosomal instability. This instability can easily lead to the production of cancerous cells.

When HPV expresses its cancer-inducing potential, it forces the infected cells to produce a set of two proteins that are the key factors in the process. When the infection takes place and the virus penetrates the nucleus of the cell where the DNA resides, it changes the DNA itself and produces a set of proteins or *building blocks* that help the virus replicate itself. It replicates quickly, revealing its aggressive nature.

The oncoproteins produced are called E6 and E7, and they are expressions of the malignant potential of HPV. The function of the E6 and E7 oncoproteins is, in fact, to extend the lifespan of the infected cells. They prevent the infected host cells from self-destructing (apoptosis), the mechanism with which the body otherwise protects itself from developing cancer. Their presence can be detected with a Pap smear and it indicates the presence of an active virus.

The E6 function binds with a receptor in the host cell, downregulating its own activity. The result of blocking the activity of the receptor is to prevent cell death. Prolonging the life of the cell provides the virus with a never-ending production of bioproducts essential to its growth and its ability to proliferate into millions of copies called *virions*.

E7 will extend the length of the *telomeres*. Telomeres are special areas of our DNA genetic material that have the function to preserve the lifespan of the cell. The telomeres are like protective caps on the ends of linear chromosomes. The length of the telomere is associated with the lifespan of the chromosome. The longer the telomere, the longer the life of the chromosome and, therefore, the longer the life of the cell. The host cells become immortal because of the viral infection.

The presence of these oncoproteins enables the infected cell itself to live and replicate indefinitely. The cell has no other choice than to be enslaved by a merciless virus. It will become immortal at the cost of promoting tumor progression and growth. The cellular process of "committing suicide" when its integrity is compromised is called *apoptosis*.

HPV IN MEN

HPV is not only a woman's concern. Men are also affected by the presence of HPV in their system, and they can be very vulnerable. There are no screening tests available for men to detect the presence of the virus. HPV is communicated via sexual contact but also through mouth-to-mouth contact, such as during a deep kiss. The virus affects men in a different way because it has the greatest affinity to growth in the oropharyngeal tract and anal area, causing mouth, throat, pharyngeal, and anal cancer.

According to the CDC data from 2007, the virus does not have the tendency to produce lesions in the male genital area and seldom causes penile cancer; the rate is as low as 0.8 per 100,000 men or 985 new cases.

Patients who are under treatment with immunosuppressant medications for health conditions—including psoriasis, asthma, ulcerative colitis, arthritis, temporal arteritis, and Crohn's disease—are at increased risk of developing serious cancer-related complications if infected with the HPV virus.

HPV PREVENTION

Regular checkups, Pap smears, and HPV testing can help detect any abnormalities early on, allowing for timely intervention and reduction of the risk for complications. Regular Pap smears and HPV testing, especially for high-risk populations, remain essential components of cervical cancer prevention and early detection efforts. These screening methods, along with vaccination against high-risk HPV types, play a crucial role in reducing the incidence and burden of cervical cancer worldwide.

It's true that using condoms can lower the risk of HPV transmission, but they do not offer complete protection. This is primarily because HPV (human papillomavirus) can be spread through skin-to-skin contact in areas not covered by a condom. HPV often infects areas of the genitals that may not be covered by a condom—e.g., the surrounding genital skin. Even with consistent and correct condom use, there is still some risk of transmission.

A vaccine is available to prevent infection with high-risk HPV in both men and women. Currently, the vaccine is mainly recommended for children ages eleven or twelve to protect them at the time of exposure to the virus through sexual contact.

The vaccine demonstrated a 64 percent decrease in the prevalence of HPV infection with types 6, 11, 16, and 18.

The quadrivalent vaccine, introduced in 2006, prevents infection from HPV with almost 100 percent efficacy. Gardasil provides protection against 80 to 90 percent of genital wart–causing HPV infections.[20] (Bonnez and Reichman, 2010; CDC, 2010a)

The vaccine also can assist in preventing penile, anal, and oral cancers due to HPV 16 and 18.

In June 2019, the Centers for Disease Control and Prevention Advisory Committee on Immunization Practices recommended vaccination based on shared clinical decision-making for individuals aged twenty-seven to forty-five years who are not adequately vaccinated.

According to the most recent data available from the U.S. Centers for Disease Control and Prevention (CDC), HPV vaccination rates among adolescents—ages thirteen through seventeen—in the United States continue to improve each year, but there is still room for growth. Key points include:

- **Overall coverage**: As of 2021 data published in 2022, about **59–62 percent** of adolescents ages thirteen through seventeen were up to date with the HPV vaccination series. "Up to date" typically means having received all recommended doses—two doses if the series is started before age fifteen, or three doses if started on or after the fifteenth birthday.

- **At least one dose**: A higher percentage—often reported between **75–80 percent**—of adolescents in the same age group have received **at least one dose** of the HPV vaccine.

These figures can vary depending on location—state-level data, demographic factors, and year-to-year changes, so the exact percentages may shift slightly in newer reports.

For the most up-to-date statistics and state-by-state breakdowns, you can visit the CDC's **National Immunization Survey – Teen (NIS-Teen)** page:

- CDC: TeenVaxView

The HPV vaccine requires three doses, and it is quite expensive to buy without insurance—about three hundred fifty dollars for each dose. Many health insurance companies cover the cost of the vaccination for patients up to age forty-five. Patients older than forty-five are not currently covered because of the lack of the FDA approval.

There are many situations in which both women and men older than forty-five, with an HPV-negative status, decide to start dating again, sometimes after a divorce.

Through a new partner, they might find themselves exposed to the risk of contracting a new infection, the HPV virus.

Managing HPV Infection, Controlling the Disease

The best way to protect our body from HPV-related complications or to promote the clearance of the virus from our system is to keep our immune system strong and efficient.

Patients who are under immunosuppressive therapy for chronic autoimmune disorders such as Crohn's disease, rheumatoid arthritis, multiple sclerosis, temporal arteritis, and psoriasis, or due to organ transplant, are at the highest risk of developing cancer from harboring HPV in their system; therefore, they should be monitored for the possibility of contracting cancer induced by the presence of HPV. HIV-positive patients are immune suppressed; therefore, they are also at very high risk of developing HPV-induced cancers.

Always talk to your medical provider about what to expect from taking an immunosuppressant while being treated for cancer. All patients receiving immunosuppressive therapy should be screened for high-risk HPV prior to initiating their treatment. Also, patients diagnosed with HPV-induced cancer and undergoing medical treatment need to know the immunosuppressant therapy to treat the comorbid conditions like Crohn's disease, ulcerative colitis, MS, or psoriasis will increase the likelihood of HPV to cause cancer in the body. The same applies to patients who are a recipient of a transplant and, therefore, taking immunosuppressant medications.

One of the first young patients to come for her routine exam to my new office on Cape Cod in 1990 had an abnormal Pap smear result for a severe precancerous lesion of her cervix, confirmed with a colposcopy. She was tested for STDs to find out that she was seropositive for HIV. She had no other symptoms of her disease, and she died of HIV-related complications shortly after, at a very young age.

Menopause increases the risk of contracting HPV infection together with other sexually transmitted diseases because of the weakening of the ability of the immune system to fight infections. In the menopausal state there is a significant decrease in the number of B-cells and CD8+ cells in the outer portion of the cervix, meaning the tissue is more prone not only to infection but also to harboring the infection for a much longer time.

Another problem is that the pace at which the cells renew and exfoliate is much slower than in younger women, leading to a persistent infection with the agent responsible.

Screening for Female Cancer

Promoting heightened awareness to empower
early cancer diagnosis and prevention

Early detection plays a pivotal role in successful cancer treatment.

In this publication, my aim is to emphasize the significance of cancer screening and prevention, shedding light on crucial topics that can empower individuals to take proactive measures against this devastating disease. By raising awareness about the benefits of early diagnosis and less invasive treatment options, medical providers strive to improve patient outcomes and overall well-being.

CANCER PREVENTION/ EARLY DIAGNOSIS

There are two modalities of cancer prevention. The first one is the *primary prevention*, aimed at removing the cause responsible for producing cancer. One example of primary prevention is to vaccinate patients against the most common oncogenic and high-risk strains of HPV, thereby decreasing the risk of contracting the infection upon exposure.

The *secondary prevention* is early diagnosis. It allows cancer to be diagnosed early in its growth when it is easier to treat and remove from the system. Mammography and Pap smears fall into the category of "screening tests" designed to establish an early diagnosis of cancer in women. One example of secondary prevention, for instance, is relative to the diagnosis of an early, noninvasive lesion in the breast discoverable by mammography.

Breast Cancer

There are different ways to screen women for cancer as well as to establish an early diagnosis. The first and most common test is the *mammogram*. Mammography is the only recognized screening test for breast cancer, although its detection rate is only about 75 percent. This means that 25 percent of cancers may go undetected.

This is especially true for a particular kind of breast cancer called *lobular cancer*. It is not unusual for some patients to find a lump on the breast a few months after a completely normal mammogram. Ultrasound of the breast will add some information about the cystic or solid nature of the lump, distinguishing between a benign cyst versus a *fibroadenoma* or a malignancy.

Ultrasound of the breast serves as a crucial adjunctive tool to mammography in enhancing the ability to diagnose any pathology of the breast tissue as well as early cancer detection.

There is another test available called *thermography*, which could aid in the screening and diagnosis of breast cancer. Thermography has a much lower detection rate compared to mammography. According to a study published in the journal *Breast Care*, the specificity for thermography is about 57.8 percent with an accuracy of 69.1 percent. (Omranipour, et al. 2016)

In October 2017, the FDA published a statement against relying only on thermography alone as a diagnostic test. The FDA clearly indicated that there is no scientific evidence to support the use of thermography as an alternative test to mammography, which remains "the most effective screening method for detecting breast cancer in its early and therefore most treatable stages." The FDA considers thermography as an "adjunctive tool" that can be used together with mammography but does not replace it.

OVARIAN/ TUBAL CANCERS EARLY DIAGNOSIS

Another category of tests available for assisting in the diagnosis of some ovarian and tubal cancers are special blood tests called *tumor markers*.

Two of these tests are available today: the Ca 125 and HE4 test.

Both these tests are not considered screening tests for ovarian cancer because they can only aid in the diagnosis of a special subset of ovarian cancer called *epithelial*.

Both tests have a high rate of false positive readings, especially in women of reproductive age, and both are more reliable in postmenopausal women.

We have made huge progress in our ability to screen for and to diagnose cancer. We are very far from having found a real cure for it.

Most of the cancer treatments currently available are mainly aimed at destroying malignant cells but are not specific for them.

Radiation and chemotherapy both target rapidly dividing cells.

In our bodies, healthy tissues—such as the intestinal lining, the immune cells, and the blood—are made of cells that divide quite rapidly.

The cancer treatment will not be able to distinguish between healthy, rapidly dividing cells and cancerous cells. The result is that treatments become both highly toxic and potentially dangerous for the entire body, with serious side effects and possible long-term complications.

Patients who receive chemo and radiation therapy become immunosuppressed because the *lymphocytes*—or immune cells responsible for protecting our bodies against parasites, viruses, bacteria—and paradoxically malignant cells are highly sensitive to the treatments. The effect of radiation and chemotherapy can also damage our DNA material, resulting in the development of secondary cancers.

The Importance of Early Diagnosis

When cancer is diagnosed in the early stages of development, there is a better chance of recovering from it with less invasive treatments. Patients should be advised of the importance of screening for cancer to establish an early diagnosis.

CHAPTER SIX

THE TRUTH BEHIND PAP SMEARS

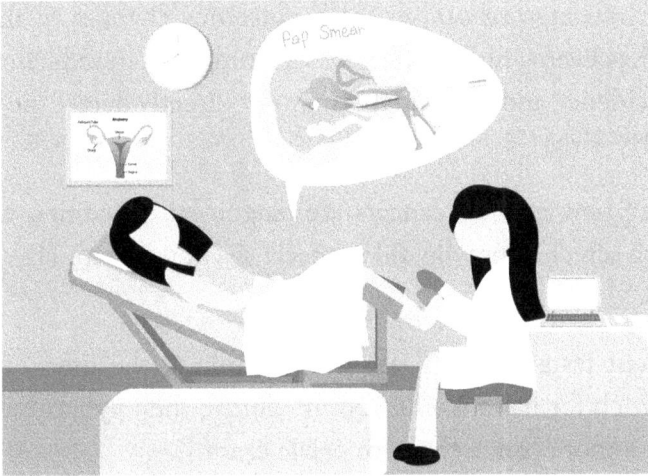

Given the widespread prevalence of HPV and its potential to cause cervical and other HPV-related cancers, regular screening and vaccination are essential preventive measures for all sexually active individuals, regardless of their relationship status. The history of a normal Pap smear in the past does not preclude the possibility of a new infection with HPV that could lead to the development of the disease. HPV infection does not cause symptoms of vaginal discharge, pain, or itching, and the only way to be diagnosed is through a specific test typically done at the time of the Pap smear.

In many circumstances, a practitioner may only request a test for HPV if the Pap smear has come back with abnormal cells. But HPV can be present in a patient with a completely normal Pap smear, and that's one of the reasons adding HPV testing at the time of the Pap smear is recommended.

Adding HPV testing to the Pap smear increases the chance of detecting severe abnormalities of the cervix by 95 percent.

Patients should request their providers to always check for their HPV status with every annual Pap smear.

The Pap smear is primarily aimed at detecting abnormal cervical cells that may indicate pre-cancerous or cancerous changes in the cervix. While it has been a highly effective screening tool in reducing cervical cancer incidence and mortality, it may not directly detect the presence of the HPV virus.

Half of all new cervical cancers are diagnosed in women who have never been screened or who did not receive a Pap smear in the previous five years.

Our current tests for HPV are done mainly at the time of the Pap smear, which for most women occurs during their gynecological visit as part of a more comprehensive pelvic exam.

A pelvic exam can reveal skin lesions of the vulva, such as melanoma or skin cancer or other abnormalities that can be present at the level of their vagina, anus, uterus, and ovaries.

The most common strains of HPV associated with the diagnosis of cervical cancer are HPV 16 and 18, which account for 70 percent of cervical cancer cases.

They are also found in 24.3 percent of women with low-grade cervical dysplasia and 51.1 percent of women diagnosed with high-grade cervical dysplasia. (WHO/ ICO 2010)

HPV 16 accounts for almost 12 percent of all cancers in women, and cervical cancer represents the second most frequent gynecological malignancy in the world.

The prognosis of cervical cancer depends on the staging of the tumor.

According to the statistics, the five-year overall survival rate is 72 percent in North America. Worldwide, 52 percent of women with cervical cancer die of the disease. (WHO/ ICO 2010)

With early detection and treatment, 80–90 percent of women with stage I cancer and 50–65 percent of women with stage II cancer are alive five years after the diagnosis.

As a result of the wrong message delivered to patients by the medical establishment, which recommends gynecological exams with Pap smears not until age twenty-one and every five years if negative for HPV, we in the U.S. now have an increase in the cases of cervical cancer in women younger than fifty.

We have 14,100 new cases of cervical cancer detected and 4280 related deaths each year in the U.S.

These recommendations seem to ignore the fact that Pap smears have a large rate of false negatives and HPV testing is only good for 10 percent of the high-risk HPV while accounting for false negative rates as well.

How the Pap Smear Evolved as a Screening Technique

The Pap smear was invented by Dr. Papanicolaou, a Greek cytologist working at Cornell University in New York State in the 1900s. He published his method in an article entitled "New Cancer Diagnosis" in 1928. Dr. Papanicolaou realized how important the screening method was to detect precancerous lesions as well as cervical cancer.

In 1952, a large clinical trial was launched of secondary prevention of cervical cancer, using Papanicolaou's smearing technique. During the study, 557 patients were found with pre-invasive cancer—early-stage, localized lesions curable by simple surgical procedures.

The average age of diagnosis was twenty years younger than the average age of women with invasive lesions, corroborating the long path of carcinogenesis. The Pap smear had, in effect, pushed the clock of cancer detection forward by nearly two decades, and it changed the spectrum of cervical cancer from predominantly incurable to predominantly curable.

There are two kinds of Pap smears available. The traditional and time-tested method involves obtaining a sample of cells from the cervix or vaginal walls, which is then smeared onto a thin glass slide, treated with a fixative, and subsequently examined under a microscope. This kind of Pap smear has a lower cost and is used largely in countries where the economy is not strong.

The second and more accepted kind of Pap smear is liquid based. The sample obtained from the cervix or vagina is placed in a vial containing a special solution. The solution with the sample is then filtered to remove blood, sperm, and other debris and placed on a very thin layer for the cytologist to review under the microscope. This technique is called *thin prep*, and it is widely in use in the U.S.

According to a large review of studies published in the medical literature, made by Cox, et al in 2004, the ability to identify abnormal cells for the thin prep Pap smear is higher than the traditional Pap smear: 81 percent versus 71 percent. (Cox 2024)

The Pap smear will detect abnormal cells derived from the cervix, uterus, and vaginal walls but also will assist in the detection of bacteria, fungi, and parasites present in the vaginal canal. Adding HPV testing to the Pap smear increases the accuracy of the result and the ability to diagnose cancer. The combination of HPV testing plus Pap smear catches twice as many cervical lesions as the Pap smear alone. (Hurtado-Salgado, et al. 2021)

Dr. Harald Zur Hausen was a German virologist who discovered the association between HPV infection and cervical cancer, winning a Nobel Prize in medicine in 2008. He was able to identify two different strains of the virus, type 16 and 18, present at the level of tissue specimens derived from cervical cancer lesions.

We now know both strains, together with HPV 9, are responsible for 81 percent of cases of cervical cancer.

HOW ACCURATE IS THE PAP SMEAR IN CANCER DETECTION?

The false negative rate for a Pap smear ranges from 20 percent to 45 percent, depending on the study. According to a study published by Dr. Yang Liu, et al. at the Department of Reproduction of Kunming Medical University in Kunming, China, the Pap smear false-negative rate is 43.2 percent. (2022). A false negative result means the test does not detect abnormalities, even though they may be present.

There are several reasons why a Pap test may produce a false negative result:

- *Quality.* The Pap test involves collecting cells from the cervix and the endo-cervical canal using a small brush or spatula. If the sample obtained is not representative of the cervix, the test may miss an abnormality.

- *Quantity.* The sample collected should contain enough cervical and endo-cervical cells.

- *Contamination.* A sample contaminated with blood or inflammation may not be as accurate as it should be. Blood, inflammatory cells, or the presence of abundant and thick mucus in the cervical canal lower the ability to detect abnormal cells.

Empower Your Health

Increased Risk of Concurrent STIs

The statistics highlight the significant impact of STIs on public health. Each year, a considerable number of new HIV cases, sexually transmitted infections (STIs), unintended pregnancies, and sexual assaults occur, underscoring the ongoing need for education, prevention, and healthcare interventions to address these issues.

Each year, an estimated 45,000 new cases of HIV and approximately 20 million sexually transmitted infections occur, three million women experience unintended pregnancies, and one million women are sexually assaulted. The Centers for Disease Control and Prevention reported a trend of increasing rates of STDs.

In the USA, data shows an incidence of HPV of thirteen million; it is the most common STD in the US.21 https://www.cdc.gov/sti/media/images/SPICE-prevalence-vs-incidence.png.

Frequency of Pap Smears and HPV Testing:

Pap smears and HPV testing should be considered in the context of individual risk factors and healthcare recommendations. While it's true that some guidelines suggest a three-to-five-year interval between Pap smears for women with normal results, this does not mean that regular screening should be disregarded or that new HPV infections cannot occur during that time.

The timing and frequency of these screenings may vary based on individual factors such as age, medical history, sexual activity, and the presence of high-risk factors. Women who have multiple sexual partners, have a history of HPV or other STIs, or have other risk factors may need more frequent screenings to detect any changes or infections promptly.

Guidelines have evolved over time to consider the most effective and evidence-based screening strategies for cervical cancer prevention. In some cases, healthcare providers may recommend co-testing—both Pap smear and HPV testing—to enhance the sensitivity of detection and improve patient outcomes, especially for those at higher risk.

Educating patients about HPV, its potential for latent infections, and the importance of regular screenings is vital for promoting better sexual health.

Open communication between patients and healthcare providers helps individuals understand their specific risk factors and receive personalized care to mitigate potential risks associated with HPV and cervical cancer.

THE CONCEPT OF A SATISFACTORY PAP SMEAR

A *satisfactory Pap smear* refers to a cervical screening test that has provided a sufficient and adequate sample of cells from the cervix for evaluation by the laboratory. When a Pap smear is deemed satisfactory, it means that the sample obtained during the procedure contains an adequate number of cells and that the cells are well-preserved and suitable for evaluation under the microscope.

A satisfactory Pap smear is essential for accurate interpretation by the pathologist or cytotechnologist. It allows them to properly assess the cervical cells for any abnormalities, including changes that may indicate precancerous or cancerous conditions, as well as other cervical or gynecological issues.

If a Pap smear is labeled as unsatisfactory due to insufficient cell sample or poor cell preservation, it may result in the need for a repeat test, as the initial sample may not provide enough information for a reliable assessment.

It is essential for healthcare providers and laboratory personnel to ensure Pap smears are conducted correctly and that the collected sample meets the criteria for being a satisfactory specimen. Regular and satisfactory Pap smears are crucial for effective cervical cancer screening and early detection of any potential abnormalities in the cervix.

The endocervical canal is an essential part of the cervix that can sometimes be challenging to sample adequately during a Pap smear. The endo-cervical canal is the space located inside the cervix, it contains glandular cells that are also susceptible to changes and abnormalities.

The ability to collect cells from the endocervical canal during a Pap smear is crucial because abnormal cells could be present deep within this canal. If these abnormal cells are not detected and treated in a timely manner, they may progress to cancer without early intervention.

Accessing the endocervical canal may be difficult due to several circumstances:

- *Anatomy and Technique.* The endocervical canal can have a complex and tortuous structure, making it a challenge to reach with standard sampling devices during a Pap smear.

- *Menopausal Changes.* In older women, hormonal changes during menopause can lead to thinning of the cervical lining—cervical atrophy. The external opening to the endo-cervix can become difficult to find and in some cases, impossible to bypass.

- *Scarring.* Scarring of the cervical tissue, which can occur due to previous cervical procedures like cone biopsy or loop electrosurgical excision procedure (LEEP) or cryotherapy, may prevent access to the endocervical canal.

- *Narrowing.* The endocervical canal can also narrow due to natural aging processes or conditions like cervical stenosis.

When the endocervical canal cannot be adequately sampled during a Pap smear, it is known as an *inadequate* or *unsatisfactory* sample.

In such cases, repeat testing or additional procedures, such as colposcopy or endocervical curettage, may be necessary to examine the area more closely and ensure proper evaluation of the cervical cells.

Healthcare providers must be aware of these challenges and consider the individual's risk factors and medical history to determine the most appropriate screening and follow-up strategies. Regular communication between patients and their healthcare providers is crucial to ensuring comprehensive cervical cancer screening and early detection of any potential abnormalities.

Sometimes practitioners encounter a clinical situation in which a patient who has undergone a surgical procedure called D&C—dilation and curettage—is diagnosed with a serious pre-cancerous lesion of the cervix that was not diagnosed at the time of her routine Pap smear.

This situation is classified as "false negative result" because the Pap smear failed to capture the abnormal cells that were hiding deeply inside her endo-cervical canal.

This situation is more common in older patients because it can be harder to retrieve cells from the endocervical.

Current screening guidelines do not recommend that women are tested annually if they have had no history of abnormal Pap smears.

I feel it is important to know with absolute certainty the Pap smear was done correctly and that it was truly representative of the patient's real condition since knowing the risk of the patient determines the frequency of the test.

It is of utmost importance to add HPV testing to every Pap smear even under negative results, even if the cells all look normal, because adding knowledge about HPV status will help to determine the cervical cancer risk status of the patient, and it will ultimately help in planning the best plan of care tailored to the patient.

There are conditions that lower the quality of the sample like the presence of abundant and thick mucus in the cervical canal or the contamination with blood and inflammatory cells.

A recent study showed that 16 percent of patients who had an unsatisfactory Pap smear have either a precancerous lesion or cancer of the cervix. A close follow-up is required when the Pap smear is not considered satisfactory. Always ask your medical provider if your Pap smear is satisfactory.

Creating a new collecting device to improve the accuracy and representation of Pap smears is a commendable initiative. Improving the sampling process can lead to better detection of abnormalities, early intervention, and ultimately better healthcare outcomes for patients.

The most common Pap-smear-collecting tools available today have significant flaws and limitations that can affect the quality of the Pap smear.

During many years of clinical practice, I have been acutely aware of the issue and its sequels. Through my experience, I recognized the need for an improved Pap smear collecting device to address the discomfort and bleeding often experienced by patients during the procedure.

This is the reason why I have designed and patented a new collecting device that can be tailored to the size and shape of the patient's cervix, addressing one of the challenges in obtaining samples from the endocervical canal effectively. Such innovation has the potential to enhance the quality of Pap smears and increase the likelihood of capturing cells from the deeper areas of the cervix, where abnormal cells might be hiding.

The ability to provide a richer and more representative sample could significantly benefit patients, as it may lead to earlier detection of abnormalities, more accurate diagnoses, and improved management strategies. Moreover, healthcare providers would have more confidence in the results, enabling them to make well-informed decisions regarding patient care.

The new Pap smear collecting device is also designed to minimize trauma to the cervix and discomfort of the patient with the exam while improving the yield of a sample obtained from the cervix. Using the new device may improve the overall experience for the patients. Less trauma also means reducing the incidence of bleeding. The presence of blood in the Pap smear sample can compromise its accuracy by obscuring the presence of abnormal cells.

The new device is in the process of going through FDA approval, and it will be available on the market soon after.

THE IMPORTANCE OF A YEARLY PELVIC EXAM

The pelvic exam is an essential component of women's healthcare and is typically performed by a gynecologist or another qualified healthcare provider. The Pap smear is only one of the tests currently done during a normal gynecological visit.

Pelvic exams are crucial for many reasons:

- *Early detection of gynecological issues.* Yearly pelvic exams allow healthcare providers to screen for and detect various gynecological and nongynecological issues early on. These may include abnormal growth, infections, skin lesions including melanoma, and other conditions that may not cause noticeable symptoms initially but can be treated more effectively if identified early.

- *Cervical cancer screening.* During a pelvic exam, a healthcare provider can perform a Pap smear to screen for cervical cancer, as discussed more thoroughly in earlier chapters.

- *Evaluation of reproductive health.* Pelvic exams enable healthcare providers to assess the health of the reproductive organs, including the uterus, ovaries, and fallopian tubes. They can identify irregularities, such as ovarian cysts, fibroids, or other conditions that may impact fertility or require medical attention.

- *Sexually transmitted infection (STI) screening.* In some cases, pelvic exams may include STI testing, depending on a woman's risk factors and sexual history. Early detection and treatment of STIs are essential for preventing complications and transmission to partners.

- *Menopause management.* For women going through menopause or perimenopause, pelvic exams can help monitor any related issues and address symptoms like vaginal dryness, discomfort, relaxation of the pelvic floor or other changes in the pelvic area.

- *General health assessment.* Pelvic exams provide an opportunity for healthcare providers to conduct a general health check of a woman's reproductive and pelvic organs. This may help identify issues or concerns that require further evaluation or treatment.

It is imperative that patients have a yearly gynecological exam, even in the later stages of their lives, as numerous cancers of the breast and the gynecological organs have the tendency to be more prevalent in women older than sixty.

Preventive care and early diagnosis of cancer are the keys to maintaining good health.

Section III

Optimize Your Immune System For Better Health

CHAPTER SEVEN

CANCER AND YOUR IMMUNE SYSTEM

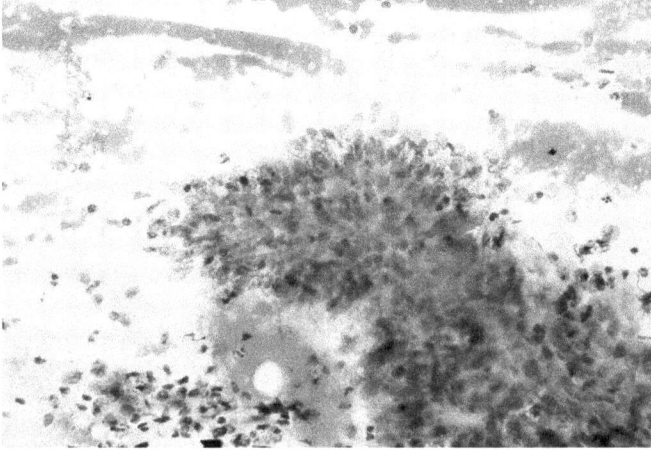

Cancer can arise due to a complex interplay of contributing factors, encompassing both genetic and environmental influences. Genetic predisposition can play a significant role, where certain inherited mutations may increase the risk of developing cancer. Environmental factors—such as exposure to carcinogens, including tobacco smoke, radiation, and harmful toxins—can trigger the initiation and progression of cancerous cells.

Lifestyle factors—such as poor nutrition, obesity, and chronic inflammatory conditions—also come into play. Furthermore, emerging research suggests that unresolved emotional issues and chronic stress might also impact cellular processes, potentially contributing to the onset of cancer.

Pathogenic factors can exert significant stress on the immune system, impairing its ability to fulfill its vital role of safeguarding the body against various threats, including cancerous cells, viruses, bacteria, and parasites found in the environment.

In summary, cancer's multifaceted nature underscores the importance of a holistic approach to prevention and early detection, addressing both genetic susceptibility and modifiable lifestyle factors to reduce the overall risk of this devastating disease.

When the immune system faces an overwhelming challenge from pathogens, it may become compromised and weakened, leaving the body more susceptible to infections, as well as allowing cancerous cells to evade immune surveillance and potentially proliferate unchecked.

By compromising the immune system's efficacy, pathogenic factors create a double-edged threat. Not only does the risk of infectious diseases increase, but the likelihood of cancer development escalates. Maintaining a robust and balanced immune response through healthy lifestyle practices, timely vaccinations, and appropriate medical interventions is essential to fortify the body's defense against both infectious agents and cancerous cells.

An unhealthy diet loaded with refined starchy foods, sugar and other sweeteners, dyes, preservatives, and processed ingredients can cause significant damage to the gastrointestinal system, weakening the integrity of its lining. Common medications such as aspirin, ibuprofen, and anti-inflammatories when taken regularly can alter the integrity of the intestinal lining as well. A damaged lining will allow toxins, pathogens, chemicals, and debris to cross over the protective layer of cells lining the intestines that act as a filter and consequently flood circulating blood, causing inflammatory changes in the body.

Inflammation is the leading cause of degenerative diseases such as arthritis, diabetes, hypertension, and obesity, and of autoimmune diseases, such as Hashimoto's thyroiditis, Multiple sclerosis (MS), Lupus erythematous, psoriasis, Crohn's disease, and ulcerative colitis.

Inflammation is a natural response of the immune system to protect the body against harmful stimuli such as pathogens or tissue damage. While acute inflammation can be beneficial in the short term by assisting in the healing process, long-term, chronic inflammation can have detrimental effects on the body leading to an increased risk of cancer and degenerative diseases.

Every minute, 200 to 300 cancer cells are spontaneously and randomly produced in our body. Every day our immune system is constantly challenged by the presence of abnormal cells with aberrant DNA material. The alteration of the DNA of the cells can also be spontaneously and randomly produced.

HOW THE BODY MEDIATES CANCER THREAT

It is up to specialized immune cells, known as *T cells*, to remove aberrant cells from circulation. When your immune system is strong and intact, it can protect your body against cancer cells, but not all cancer cells are born equal. Some have an intrinsic ability to overcome being recognized by immune cells.

Cancer cells can escape immune surveillance in several ways:

- *Displaying altered surface proteins.* Cancer cells may display different proteins on their surface, thereby escaping detection as abnormal or foreign.

- *Suppressing immune activity.* Cancer cells can secrete substances to dampen the immune response or promote an environment that inhibits immune cell activity.

- *Generating genetic instability.* The genetic instability of cancer cells can lead to rapid changes in their genetic makeup, allowing them to adapt and evade immune responses.

- *Counteracting natural apoptosis or cell death.* Cancer cells may, in fact, acquire mutations that allow them to survive and continue replicating.

The rapid reproduction and multiplication of cancer cells can be overwhelming for the immune system, leading to a decreased efficiency in the process of identifying and clearing these abnormal cells from the body.

Let me explain the process in more detail: When cancer cells proliferate at a high rate, they create a larger population of cells that the immune system needs to recognize and target for destruction. Normally, the immune system has mechanisms in place to detect and eliminate abnormal or cancerous cells. Immune cells, such as T cells and natural *killer cells*, are responsible for recognizing and destroying these cells. They do so by recognizing specific molecules, called *antigens*, present on the surface of cancer cells.

However, the rapid growth of cancer cells can lead to several challenges for the immune system. Firstly, the sheer number of cancer cells can be overwhelming, making it difficult for the immune system to keep up with their identification. This increased workload can strain the immune system's resources and reduce its efficiency in recognizing all the abnormal cells.

Secondly, cancer cells can undergo genetic changes that alter their antigenic profile. These changes can result in the production of new antigens or the loss of antigens that the immune system previously recognized. As a result, the immune system may fail to identify these altered cancer cells as threats, allowing them to escape detection and to continue proliferating.

Furthermore, cancer cells can develop various strategies to evade immune surveillance. They can produce molecules that suppress immune responses, create an immunosuppressive microenvironment around the tumor, or manipulate immune checkpoints to prevent an effective immune response. These mechanisms hinder the immune system's ability to effectively target and eliminate cancer cells.

The faster the reproduction and multiplication of cancer cells, the greater the burden on the immune system. Understanding these challenges is crucial in developing effective cancer treatments that can enhance the immune system's ability to fight cancer.

Some malignant cells can turn into perfectly engineered killing machines, most efficient in their ability to overcome the immune system.

For cancer to be successful it requires two factors:

1. A defective or weakened immune system that fails to recognize and destroy the cancerous cells.

2. A selected population of cancerous cells that expresses the ability to evade recognition from the immune system.

The combination of these two factors will produce a "perfect storm" with deadly consequences for the host. The body affected by cancer will succumb to the tyranny of the high-energetic requirements needed for the cancer's own survival and reproduction. Such a high demand will soon exhaust the natural resources of the body, leading to death.

The Connection to HPV

Oncogenic HPV is a typical example in which the host is overwhelmed by the cancer induced by the viral infection. As discussed in more detail in Chapter Five, HPV mediates cancer-inducing activity expressing the two key proteins E6 and E7. Both proteins are synthesized in the infected cell under the instruction of the virus that can interact with the DNA at the level of the nucleus.

Once released in the cells, these proteins can affect the ability of the host cell to undergo programmed apoptosis. However, certain proteins can interfere with this process and prevent the cell from undergoing apoptosis, even when its integrity is compromised. These proteins play a role in regulating apoptosis and can prevent cells from undergoing programmed cell death.

When overexpressed or present in excessive amounts, both can interfere with the normal apoptotic pathways, enabling the survival of infected cells. Therefore, the viral proteins E6 and E7 not only interfere with the host cell's self-regulating mechanisms but also provide the infected cell with the ability to continuously survive and reproduce.

This remarkable phenomenon grants the infected cell a state of *immortality* by effectively maintaining the length of telomeres within the cell. By hijacking essential cellular processes, E6 and E7 proteins counteract the normal checks and balances that would typically limit the lifespan of a cell. As explained in Chapter Five, telomeres are protective caps at the ends of chromosomes, playing a crucial role in cellular aging. With each cell division, telomeres gradually shorten, eventually triggering cell senescence or programmed cell death (apoptosis). However, the E6 and E7 proteins disrupt this natural aging process by preserving the telomere length.

The intricate mechanism employed by these viral proteins involves multiple steps. E6 interferes with the cell's tumor suppressor protein, preventing it from triggering cell death or growth arrest. This action allows the infected cell to evade apoptosis and continue to replicate.

Meanwhile, E7 disrupts the function of the retinoblastoma protein (pRb), which typically regulates cell cycle progression and prevents excessive cell division. By inactivating pRb, E7 facilitates uncontrolled cell proliferation. Furthermore, E6 and E7 work together to sustain telomere length. E6 assists in the activation of telomerase, ensuring its continuous activity and preventing telomere attrition. E7, on the other hand, promotes the synthesis of telomerase, further enhancing the preservation of telomeres.

Telomeres are typically maintained by an enzyme called *telomerase*, which adds DNA sequences to the ends of chromosomes to counteract the telomere shortening during cell division.

Understanding the mechanisms behind E6- and E7-mediated immortalization is crucial for developing effective antiviral strategies and combating viral-associated diseases, particularly those linked to HPV infection where these proteins play a central role. By targeting E6 and E7 or interfering with their interactions with host cell factors, it may be possible to disrupt the viral-mediated immortality and restore normal cell function, ultimately providing new avenues for therapeutic interventions.

It is widely accepted by the medical community that a high level of chromosome instability and DNA damage in the cell increases the risk of developing a malignancy.

"Genetic heterogeneity derived from chromosomal structural instability allows the selection of cells better adapted to their environment, which supposedly facilitates generation and progression of cancer."[22] (https:// pubmed.ncbi.nlm.nih.gov/27345585)

The cancerous process imposes significant metabolic demands on the body, gradually and inexorably siphoning away life's essence. This gradual depletion erodes the patient's strength and resilience, making even the simplest tasks daunting challenges. The relentless toll that cancer takes on the body can create an intense longing for release from the burden of suffering, as the patient's quality of life diminishes and hope wanes.

Supportive care and palliative measures play a crucial role in enhancing the patient's comfort and easing their distress during this difficult time. Empathy, compassion, and understanding are essential in providing solace and dignity for those who face the profound struggle against cancer.

As a physician intimately acquainted with the journey of caring for a lengthy roster of patients affected by cancer, and as a daughter who bore witness to the anguish and ultimate demise of her own mother who bravely faced one of the most devastating and aggressive forms of this disease, the experience has been both profoundly impactful and heart-wrenching.

Throughout my medical career, I have come face to face with the relentless nature of cancer and the toll it takes on individuals and their families. Witnessing the suffering, fear, and uncertainty that cancer brings has only strengthened my resolve to provide the best possible care and support for my patients, emphasizing not only medical expertise but also empathy and compassion.

On a deep personal level, losing my mother to cancer has been a deeply painful journey. It has given me a unique perspective on the emotional and psychological aspects that accompany this arduous battle. The devastating effects of cancer on the body and the soul are seared into my memory, fueling my commitment to making a difference in the lives of those facing similar challenges.

Through these experiences, I have grown more determined to advocate for research, early detection, and improved treatments that can offer hope and relief to those grappling with this formidable adversary. It is my sincere hope that through our collective efforts we can continue to progress in the fight against cancer, supporting patients and their families and striving toward a future in which this disease can be better controlled, if not cured entirely.

WHERE IS THE CURE?

I believe we are so far from finding the cure for cancer because we have failed to look in the right direction. In fact, it is crucial to find more targeted and specific ways to treat cancer.

Traditional treatments like chemotherapy and radiation therapy do not discriminate between cancerous and healthy cells, such as those found in the bone marrow and the gastrointestinal tract. Healthy cells in these areas naturally have a high turnover to meet the physiological demands of the body. Consequently, the nonspecific nature of radiation and chemotherapy leads to significant toxicity to the overall body.

Most common side effects of both treatments are short term, but some changes are irreversible:

- *Chemotherapy* can cause severe anemia with fatigue and a low white blood cell count, weakening the immune system.

- *Alopecia*, or diffuse hair loss, is one of the most common side effects of some chemotherapeutic agents.

- *Mutation and permanent alteration.* Radiation therapy is typically applied to the affected area of the body and can cause permanent alteration of the lining of the lungs, intestines, and heart, which can lead to severe disability. It can alter organs' functions. It can also generate secondary cancer, typically of the blood. Radiation and chemotherapy can cause serious mutation of your DNA material, resulting in the development of secondary cancers such as lymphomas induced by the treatment.

By focusing on targeted therapies and individualized treatment plans, the medical community aims to enhance the effectiveness of cancer treatments while minimizing the harm to healthy tissues. Ongoing advancements in research and technology hold great promises for improving the overall outcome and quality of life for cancer patients in the future.

To improve cancer treatments, researchers and medical professionals are actively exploring and developing more targeted and precise therapies. These newer approaches aim to distinguish between cancerous cells and healthy cells, reducing the adverse effects on the body. Examples of such targeted treatments include immunotherapy, which harnesses the body's immune system to recognize and attack cancer cells, as well as targeted therapies that focus on specific genetic mutations or proteins present in cancer cells.

New treatment modalities are available, such as:

- *Immunotherapy.* This approach harnesses the power of the immune system to target cancer cells while sparing normal cells. Immunotherapy drugs can enhance the immune response against cancer cells or remove the brakes on the immune system, allowing it to recognize and attack cancer cells more effectively.

- *Targeted therapy.* Targeted therapies focus on specific molecular changes that occur in cancer cells. By identifying the genetic mutations or abnormalities unique to cancer cells, researchers can develop drugs that specifically target these changes. This approach helps minimize harm to healthy cells and tissues.

- *Precision medicine.* Precision medicine aims to personalize cancer treatment based on an individual's specific genetic profile. By analyzing a patient's genes, practitioners can identify specific mutations or biomarkers that drive the growth of their cancer. This information can guide the selection of treatments that are most likely to be effective for that patient.

- *Nanotechnology.* Nanotechnology offers innovative solutions for targeted drug delivery. By encapsulating chemotherapy drugs or other treatment agents within nanoparticles, researchers can enhance drug accumulation in cancer cells while reducing exposure to healthy cells. This approach can potentially improve treatment efficacy and minimize side effects.

- *Gene editing.* Technologies like CRISPR-Cas9 have revolutionized gene editing, enabling scientists to make precise modifications to the genome. Researchers are exploring the use of gene editing to target cancer-causing genes or modify cancer cells to make them more susceptible to treatment.

These are just a few examples of the many promising avenues being pursued in cancer research. The goal is to develop therapies that are not only effective but also minimize harm to healthy cells and tissues. By focusing on targeted and specific approaches, researchers are striving to improve cancer treatment outcomes and ultimately find a cure.

A DIFFERENT PERSPECTIVE ON CANCER

As an OB/GYN doctor, I have always been fascinated by the remarkable similarity between early pregnancy implantation and the cancerous process.

It is truly astonishing to witness how pregnancy can successfully establish in the body, considering it represents a *foreign entity* to some extent.

During conception, when the egg is fertilized by the sperm, the resulting embryo contains 50 percent of its genetic material from the father.

This genetic makeup may not be entirely compatible with the host's body, as it carries a unique combination of genes from both parents.

Despite this inherent difference, the process of implantation involves intricate interactions between the embryo and the maternal body, which enables successful attachment and development.

The implantation process in early pregnancy shares similarities with the mechanisms that underlie tumor invasion during cancer. Both processes require complex interactions between cells and tissues, involving factors such as cell adhesion, angiogenesis—formation of new blood vessels, and immune modulation. However, there are essential differences between these processes as well.

In pregnancy, the maternal immune system plays a crucial role in accepting the semi-allogenic embryo carrying paternal genetic material and not rejecting it as a foreign entity.

On the other hand, cancer cells exploit certain mechanisms that resemble aspects of embryonic development to grow and invade tissues. They can manipulate cell signaling pathways, promoting uncontrolled proliferation and evading the immune system's surveillance.

Understanding the similarities and differences between these processes can provide valuable insights into both reproductive biology and cancer biology. Moreover, it highlights the intricacies of the human body's ability to modulate responses to diverse challenges, including the acceptance of new life and the detection and elimination of abnormal cells.

Continual research in these areas holds great potential for advancing medical knowledge and developing novel therapeutic approaches for various conditions, including infertility and cancer.

As a medical professional, I find it truly inspiring to witness how nature has evolved such complex yet finely tuned mechanisms to ensure the continuity of life. Pregnancy outcome gives birth to a healthy baby, whereas cancer's ultimate outcome is to generate chaos leading to death and destruction.

What do the two have in common?

I believe the answer could be found in the ability of both a healthy pregnancy and a *successful* cancerous process to evade recognition from the immune cells.

As a passionate OB/GYN doctor, the intriguing similarities between early pregnancy implantation and cancer processes have motivated me to undertake a research study aimed at shedding light on a crucial aspect of this phenomenon.

The main objective of my study is to identify a potential factor, secreted by the *trophoblast*—the outer layer of the early embryo—which acts in early pregnancy. This factor may possess the unique property of binding to receptors on immune cells, thereby interfering with their function and hindering their ability to recognize the trophoblast as a foreign entity.

I name the substance in question the *genesis factor*, which is essential for the successful development and growth of a pregnancy. Without this factor, a pregnancy will not be able to thrive and progress as it should.

This critical element plays a fundamental role in initiating and sustaining the complex biological processes required for the formation of a new life within the womb. It is truly the cornerstone of the beginning stages of life, and its presence is indispensable for a healthy and viable pregnancy.

Role of the Immune System in Preventing Cancer

Maintaining a healthy and robust immune system is crucial for increasing the likelihood of effectively combating HPV infection. A strong immune system can aid in clearing the virus from the body or controlling the disease, preventing its progression over time.

It is also true that a strong immune system functioning effectively can help prevent diseases caused by other pathogenic factors, such as bacteria, parasites, and other dangerous viruses, and to isolate and destroy abnormal and cancerous cells that randomly emerge in the body because of the interaction with the environment.

Cigarette and cigar smoking, for instance, can cause an increased risk of mouth, cervix, lung, and bladder cancers due to the carcinogenic effect of the toxic chemicals released in people's systems from smoking.

Certain substances, such as heavy metals, dyes, preservatives, fertilizers, and genetically modified organisms (GMOs) found in our food and environment can have potential carcinogenic effects on our bodies. They can induce damage to our DNA, the genetic blueprint of our cells, and trigger inflammatory responses that may weaken our immune system function.

- *Heavy Metals.* Heavy metals like lead, arsenic, cadmium, and mercury are toxic and can accumulate in the body over time. They have been linked to various health issues, including cancer, as they can damage cellular structures and disrupt essential biological processes.

- *Dyes and Preservatives.* Some synthetic dyes and food preservatives have been associated with adverse health effects. Certain dyes, like azo dyes, have been shown to generate harmful byproducts when metabolized in the body, potentially contributing to DNA damage and cancer risk.

- *Fertilizers.* Certain synthetic fertilizers used in industrial agriculture, as well as home gardens and yards, may contain harmful chemicals that can seep into the soil and water supply, potentially contaminating the food we consume and the places we recreate. Long-term exposure to these chemicals can be carcinogenic.

In the oceans, we are witnessing a recent and concerning phenomenon known as *red algae blooms* or *red tide*, and scientists hypothesize that one possible cause could be the spillage of fertilizers into watersheds that run down to the sea. An overabundance of nutrients like nitrogen and phosphorus flow off agricultural land and into the waterways, promoting the concentration and rapid growth of these toxic algae once they hit the ocean.

As the algae multiply, they form dense and visible patches on the water's surface, giving it a reddish or brownish hue. The overgrowth of algae consumes a large amount of oxygen in the water, leading to a significant decrease in oxygen levels. This decrease in dissolved oxygen can have devastating consequences for marine life.

The reduced oxygen concentration in the water creates what is called *hypoxia* or *dead zones*. In these areas, oxygen levels are insufficient to support the survival of many marine organisms. As a result, fish, shellfish, and other aquatic fauna in the affected regions suffocate and die. The lack of oxygen also disrupts the ecosystem's balance, as some species may be more tolerant of low oxygen levels, leading to imbalances in predator-prey relationships.

The death of marine fauna on such a massive scale has severe repercussions on the entire marine ecosystem, including fish populations, seabirds, marine mammals, and other organisms dependent on these resources. Furthermore, these toxic algal blooms can produce harmful toxins that may pose a risk to human health when contaminated seafood is consumed.

The occurrence of red algae blooms is a serious environmental concern that requires immediate attention. Preventing excessive fertilizer runoff, improving waste management practices, and raising awareness about the environmental impact of human activities are some of the steps that can be taken to mitigate the frequency and intensity of these harmful algal blooms. It is essential to safeguard the health of our oceans and the diverse life it sustains for the well-being of our planet and future generations.

- *GMO Foods.* Genetically modified organisms result from alterations to their DNA to achieve specific traits, such as pest resistance or improved nutritional content. While GMO foods are generally considered safe for consumption, some studies suggest they might have unforeseen health risks, including possible carcinogenic effects. More research is needed to fully understand their long-term impact on human health.

- *Carcinogenesis and Inflammation.* Exposure to these harmful substances can lead to the production of reactive oxygen species and free radicals, causing oxidative stress and inflammation in the body. Chronic inflammation is associated with an increased risk of cancer development, as it can disrupt normal cellular processes and promote tumor growth.

- *Weakened Immune System.* Prolonged exposure to carcinogenic substances and chronic inflammation can suppress the immune system's ability to identify and eliminate cancerous cells. A weakened immune system might fail to recognize and attack cancer cells effectively, allowing them to grow and spread.

To keep the body healthy while minimizing potential risks, it is essential to adopt a balanced and varied diet, limit exposure to harmful substances, and ensure food safety through proper handling and sourcing. Government regulations and oversight of food and environmental safety are also crucial to protect public health. Additionally, ongoing scientific research is necessary to better understand the potential risks associated with these substances and develop appropriate preventive measures.

How Diet Impacts Your Health

Diet plays an important role in the way your brain and body function. What I refer to as a *wrong diet*—one rich in sugar, processed food, and genetically modified food—causes increased inflammation in the body, accelerating the aging process and increasing the chance of developing conditions such as hypertension, diabetes, arthritis, Alzheimer's, cancer, and autoimmune diseases such as rheumatoid arthritis, lupus, and Hashimoto's disease.

Inflammatory changes in the body can also modify the way genes are expressed in the DNA, increasing the risk of mutations and, ultimately, cancer. Most of us understand how important it is to follow a diet rich in fresh, organic vegetables; some fresh fruit; and meats from grass-fed and free-ranging animals; and to cut down on milk and dairy as well as processed food.

Our children are at the highest risk of obesity and inflammatory changes in their bodies that can lead to premature aging and diseases. We need to ban unhealthy processed grains and other processed foods, preservatives, sweeteners, food additives, food dyes, excessively milled products, meat derived from animals fed with unhealthy processed grains, GMO food, excessive amounts of saturated fat, and sugar. The "American diet" is full of these unhealthy elements.

The most affordable food options often consist of the unhealthiest list of ingredients, including refined sugar, corn syrup, excessive salt, and preservatives, while offering the least nutritional value. Lower-cost processed and fast foods frequently contain high amounts of refined sugar and corn syrup, which contribute to empty calories without providing essential nutrients. These added sugars can lead to weight gain, obesity, and an increased risk of chronic health conditions like type 2 diabetes and heart disease.

Additionally, cheap foods tend to be laden with excessive salt to enhance flavor and extend shelf life. High salt intake is linked to hypertension and cardiovascular problems, posing serious health risks. Furthermore, many inexpensive food products contain preservatives to prolong their shelf life and maintain appearance. While these additives help extend the product's longevity, they offer little to no nutritional benefits and may have adverse health effects when consumed in excess.

Due to their low production costs and high availability, these unhealthy and nutrient-poor foods are often the most accessible options for individuals on tight budgets. Unfortunately, reliance on such foods can lead to inadequate intake of essential vitamins, minerals, and other nutrients necessary for maintaining good health and preventing malnutrition.

In contrast, healthier and more nutritious foods, such as fresh fruits, vegetables, whole grains, lean proteins, and unprocessed foods, can be more expensive, making them less accessible to individuals with limited financial resources. This economic barrier often contributes to disparities in nutrition and health outcomes between different socioeconomic groups.

Efforts to promote better nutrition and public health should include initiatives to make healthier foods more affordable and accessible to all segments of society. Policies focused on subsidizing and incentivizing the production and consumption of nutritious foods can play a crucial role in improving the overall health and well-being of the population, regardless of their income levels.

CHAPTER EIGHT

SUPPLEMENTS MAKE A DIFFERENCE

There are several over-the-counter (OTC) supplements that are believed to assist the immune system. It's important to note that while these supplements may have some supportive effects on the immune system, they should not be considered a replacement for a healthy lifestyle, balanced diet, and proper medical care when necessary.

VITAMINS

Vitamin A

- *Protection of the cervix*. Often referred to as the *anticancer vitamin*, vitamin A plays a crucial role in protecting cervical tissue against the activity of HPV. Its functions include safeguarding the integrity of the epithelial barrier from infection and activating immune cells like *phagocytes* and *cytotoxic T cells*, which help combat HPV infections.

- The risk for HPV persistence doubled with low levels of vitamin A and *lycopene*, the plant nutrient that gives tomatoes and other foods their red-orange coloring—due to the antioxidant activity of these nutrients. Antioxidant activity is also important in controlling the viral load and proliferation.

- *Anti-tumor*. Additionally, vitamin A has been found to possess tumor-inhibiting properties, making it valuable in preventing potential tumor development and progression.

- *Antioxidant.* Furthermore, vitamin A exhibits antioxidant abilities, effectively neutralizing harmful free radicals and protecting cells from oxidative damage.

- *Brain and eye health.* Beyond its anticancer effects, vitamin A is essential for maintaining brain and eye health. It supports optimal brain function and contributes to good vision, particularly in low-light conditions. Adequate vitamin A intake is essential for overall visual performance.

Here's a quick list of foods that are rich in **Vitamin A:**

- **Liver** (beef, chicken, or pork)

- **Sweet Potatoes**

- **Carrots**

- **Dark Leafy Greens** (spinach, kale, collard greens)

- **Butternut Squash**

- **Pumpkin**

- **Cantaloupe**

- **Mangoes**

- **Eggs**

- **Fortified Dairy Products** (milk, cheese)

- **Red Bell Peppers**

- **Dried Apricots**

Additional Information:

- **Preformed Vitamin A (Retinol)**: Found in animal-based foods like liver, dairy products, and eggs.

- **Provitamin A (Beta-Carotene)**: Found in plant-based sources such as carrots, sweet potatoes, and leafy greens. The body converts beta-carotene into active vitamin A as needed.

Tips:

- Including a variety of both animal- and plant-based sources can help ensure adequate vitamin A intake.

- Cooking can enhance the absorption of beta-carotene from plant sources. For example, adding a small amount of healthy fat—like olive oil—when cooking vegetables can improve absorption.

In summary, ensuring sufficient intake of vitamins or supplements can promote optimal health and help prevent certain diseases.

Vitamin B9

Folate, also known as *vitamin B9*, is a crucial nutrient responsible for maintaining the integrity of the genome and playing a vital role in gene expression regulation. *Folic acid*, a synthetic form of folate, has demonstrated a protective effect against certain cancers, among them colorectal and breast cancer. Folic acid has been associated with a significant 40 percent reduction in the rate of these cancers.[23] (https://ajcn.nutrition.org/article/S0002-9165(22)03668-1/fulltext)

Additionally, folate administration before the existence of pre-neoplastic lesions can play a preventive role in tumor development. Ensuring adequate folate levels may potentially hinder the progression of pre-cancerous cells into full-blown tumors.

Vitamin C

Also known as *ascorbic acid*, vitamin C plays a crucial role in maintaining overall health and well-being. Its importance lies in how it supports various aspects of our body's functioning:

- *Immune System Support.* Vitamin C is essential for supporting a robust immune system, helping to strengthen the body's natural defenses against infections and illnesses.

- *Nutrient Absorption.* It aids in the absorption of important nutrients such as iron from the diet, ensuring better utilization by the body.

- *Skin Health.* Vitamin C promotes the production of collagen, a vital protein for maintaining healthy and youthful skin, thereby contributing to skin health.

- *Antioxidant Properties.* As a powerful antioxidant, vitamin C helps protect the body's cells from oxidative stress caused by free radicals, making it one of the most important anti-aging substances in the body.

- *Anticarcinogenic Potential.* Its antioxidant activity also enables vitamin C to detoxify carcinogens and hinder carcinogenic processes, potentially reducing the risk of certain cancers.

- *Anti-hypertensive Effects.* Vitamin C has been associated with blood pressure regulation, contributing to a potential reduction in hypertension risks.

- *Antiviral Benefits.* It exhibits antiviral properties that can support the body's defense against certain viral infections.

- *Immunomodulatory Actions.* Vitamin C can influence and regulate the immune system, further supporting overall immune function.

In summary, vitamin C's multifaceted benefits make it a vital component in maintaining good health, promoting a strong immune system, supporting nutrient absorption, preserving skin health, and exhibiting various protective properties against aging, cancer, and certain diseases. Including vitamin C-rich foods—such as fresh fruit, sweet potatoes, and fresh, minimally processed vegetables—or supplements in the diet is an essential way to harness its numerous health advantages.

Vitamin D

A study published in the *Journal of the National Cancer Institute* in 2019 found that higher doses of 25-hydroxy vitamin D were inversely associated with the risk of colorectal cancer. In other words, increased levels of vitamin D were linked to a decreased risk of developing colorectal cancer. Study shows that higher doses of 25 hydroxy vitamin D are inversely associated with the risk of colorectal cancer. (McCollough, et al. 2019)

According to research conducted by Braun, et al., higher levels of vitamins are associated with reduced mortality and morbidity in cancer patients. This suggests that cancer patients with higher vitamin levels may experience better outcomes and a lower risk of complications. High levels of vitamins are associated with a decrease in mortality and morbidity in cancer patients.[24] (https://www.annalsofoncology.org/article/S0923-7534(21)01993-1/fulltext)

A study published in the *Critical Journal of Medicine* in 2012 reported that individuals with low levels of serum 25-hydroxy vitamin D were associated with increased mortality. In simpler terms, lower vitamin D levels were linked to a higher risk of death.[25] (https://pubmed.ncbi.nlm.nih.gov/33553987)

Overall, ensuring sufficient vitamin D intake through diet, supplements, or exposure to sunlight may be beneficial for overall health and disease prevention.

Vitamin E

Fat-soluble vitamins, such as vitamin E, and *essential minerals*, such as selenium and zinc, decrease total mortality and increase the resistance to infections, playing an important role in the maintenance of the immune system. Zinc must be present in the diet to better utilize the vitamin E in the body.

Vitamin E has many immune-regulating properties:

- *Immune System Support.* Vitamin E acts as an immune regulator, meaning it helps to modulate and balance the immune response. It supports the proper functioning of various components of the immune system.

- *White Blood Cell Production.* The thymus and spleen are essential organs for immune function. Vitamin E stimulates the production of white blood cells, particularly T cells, in the thymus and spleen. T cells play a central role in the immune response by recognizing and targeting foreign invaders, such as bacteria, viruses, and other pathogens.

- *Intestinal Mucosa Protection.* Vitamin E plays a vital role in maintaining the health and integrity of the intestinal mucosa, which lines the inner walls of the gut. This mucosal layer acts as a semipermeable layer, preventing the migration of harmful bacteria and other potentially harmful substances from the gut into the bloodstream while allowing nourishing substances to pass through. When the intestinal mucosa becomes compromised, a condition known as *leaky gut syndrome* can develop. In leaky gut syndrome, toxins, bacteria, and undigested food particles pass through the defective gut wall and enter the bloodstream. This can lead to inflammation and may contribute to various health issues.

- *Antioxidant Properties.* Vitamin E is a potent antioxidant, protecting cells and tissues from oxidative damage caused by free radicals. Free radicals are highly reactive molecules that can cause cellular damage, leading to inflammation and immune system impairment. By neutralizing these free radicals, vitamin E helps reduce oxidative stress and supports the immune system's ability to function optimally.

In summary, ensuring adequate intake of vitamin E through a balanced diet or supplements can contribute to a robust and balanced immune response, helping the body defend against infections and maintain optimal health.

OTHER HELPFUL NUTRIENTS

Astragalus

Astragalus, also known as *Huang-qi* or the *Yellow Leader*, is a perennial plant whose root has been used in traditional Chinese medicine for centuries for a variety of purposes.

- *Immunostimulant Properties.* Astragalus stimulates various components of the immune system, such as *macrophages*, which are immune cells that play a crucial role in engulfing and eliminating harmful pathogens and foreign substances.

- *Antibody Formation.* Astragalus promotes the formation of antibodies, which are essential for recognizing and neutralizing specific antigens—foreign invaders—in the body. This antibody formation is crucial for strong immune defense. It also stimulates a higher level of interferon production. Interferons are a group of cytokines that possess potent antiviral and anti-cancer properties, further bolstering the body's defense mechanisms.

- *T-Lymphocytes Proliferation*. T-lymphocytes, a type of white blood cell, are critical for coordinating the immune response and attacking infected or cancerous cells. Astragalus can increase the proliferation of T-lymphocytes, enhancing their effectiveness in combating infections and potentially inhibiting tumor growth.

- *Antioxidant Properties*. Astragalus contains potent antioxidants that help neutralize harmful free radicals in the body. By reducing oxidative stress and cellular damage caused by free radicals, astragalus contributes to overall health and may help protect against chronic diseases.

- *Antiviral effects*. Studies have shown that astragalus has antiviral properties, making it effective in inhibiting the replication of certain viruses. This can be beneficial in supporting the body's defense against viral infections.

- *Hepatoprotective effects*. Astragalus has been found to have hepatoprotective properties, meaning it can help protect the liver from damage and support its proper functioning. This is particularly important in maintaining overall health, as the liver plays a central role in detoxification and metabolism.

- *Cardiotonic effects*. Astragalus has been traditionally used as a cardiotonic herb, meaning it can strengthen and support the heart's function. It may have beneficial effects on cardiovascular health and contribute to maintaining a healthy heart.

- *Anticancer Activity.* Astragalus has shown vigorous anticancer activity. It can potentiate the killing of tumor cells, making it a promising natural agent for cancer treatment or prevention.

- *Tonic Herb.* Astragalus is revered as a tonic herb, known for its ability to increase vital and protective energy—qi or chi—in the body, combatting fatigue and enhancing resistance to diseases. Regular use of astragalus can promote overall well-being and vitality.

- *Adaptogen.* Astragalus is classified as an adaptogen, meaning it can help the body adapt to stress and support the immune system. By acting as an adaptogen, astragalus shields the immune system from the harmful effects of stress.

- *Glucose Metabolism.* Astragalus has been found to improve glucose metabolism, making it beneficial in managing pre-diabetic or diabetic conditions. By supporting better glucose regulation, astragalus may help maintain stable blood sugar levels and contribute to overall metabolic health.

Overall, astragalus can be taken as a supplement or used in traditional herbal formulations to support overall well-being and boost the body's immune response. However, it is essential to consult with a healthcare professional before using astragalus or any herbal supplement, especially if you are pregnant, nursing, or taking other medications, to ensure it is safe and appropriate for your individual health needs.

The Importance of Maintaining a Healthy Vaginal Microenvironment:

A recent study published in the *American Journal of OB/GYN* shows that there is an association between an altered vaginal flora defined as a deviation from the typical lactobacillus-dominant bacterial environment and an increased susceptibility to HPV infection and the potential for cancer induced by the virus. HPV was found to be persistent in women with altered vaginal flora.[26] (https://pmc.ncbi. nlm.nih.gov/articles/PMC5088670)

Recent studies also indicate that being affected by bacterial vaginosis, which is one of the most common bacterial infections in women, increases the risk of contracting an infection with HPV.[27] (https:// pubmed.ncbi.nlm.nih.gov/21223574)

Probiotics

Probiotics can potentially improve vaginal health by restoring the levels of lactobacillus in vaginal secretions. Lactobacillus plays a protective role against both vaginal infections and the harmful effects of HPV.

Estrogen and Glycogen

The presence of *estrogen* in the body is essential for maintaining vaginal tissue and providing a crucial substrate called *glycogen*. Glycogen supports the survival of lactobacilli in the vaginal canal.

After menopause, decreased estrogen levels can lead to insufficient glycogen and make postmenopausal patients more susceptible to harmful bacteria overgrowth. This imbalance can cause alterations in the vaginal microbiome and pH levels, potentially leading to health issues.

Iodine

Iodine is an essential element for humans with a vital role in the production of various hormones in the body. It possesses potent antiviral, antibacterial, and anti-fungal properties.

Its protective activity extends to important glands like the thyroid, ovaries, prostate, and breasts. A deficiency in iodine can leave these glands vulnerable to diseases and impaired conditions.

Research has linked low iodine intake to an increased risk of fibrocystic diseases of the breast in women, highlighting its significance in maintaining breast health. Furthermore, iodine is a crucial antioxidant and apoptosis-inducer, making it effective against tumors and atherosclerosis. Supplementing iodine can enhance antioxidant activity and boost immune system function.

In the United States, the average iodine intake is significantly lower at 240 micrograms per day compared to Japan, where individuals consume more than 12,000 micrograms daily due to their diet rich in seaweed and seafood.

Compounding the issue, the use of added chemicals, such as perchlorate, nitrate, thiocyanate, bromine, and fluorine in our food and environment, can block the absorption of this essential element, further impacting overall iodine levels in the population.

To support optimal health and prevent deficiencies, ensuring adequate iodine intake and avoiding factors that hinder its absorption become essential. Supplementing iodine can be beneficial, particularly in regions with lower iodine intake.

Mushrooms, Lichens, and Fungus

Mushrooms such as rishi are all-important in assisting our immune system in performing at its highest level.

A Rich and Varied Diet

Patients who eat plenty of *vegetables* may have a better chance of avoiding or clearing the infection with HPV. The vitamins, fibers, and mineral contents present in them might improve the functioning of the immune system while removing toxins from the human body.

Identifying Nutritional Deficiencies:

In addition to supporting the immune system through a targeted line of supplements to fight HPV infection, we must address any nutritional imbalances that may weaken the body's defenses. Factors such as heavy metal exposure, parasites, or microbial imbalances can have a negative impact on overall health and body functioning.

To identify and address such imbalances, I have been offering a nutritional test provided by a company called "Cell-Wellbeing."

This test is designed to assess the presence of nutritional deficiencies or toxicities in the body.

It works by providing "epigenetic mapping," which is a digital scanning process that measures the frequencies emitted by four hair follicles.

It has the ability of capturing over 800 underlying indicators that can reveal the body's biological stressors. This technology focuses on prevention rather than cure. For example, nutrient demands or deficiencies may indicate gut stress, cardiovascular stress, or immune deficiencies well before any symptoms manifest.

By pinpointing any nutritional imbalances or toxicities, we can take targeted and appropriate measures to address and correct these issues. The Cell-Wellbeing test serves as a powerful tool in promoting and maintaining the health and optimal performance of the body.

By combining immune support through supplements and addressing nutritional imbalances, we aim to provide a comprehensive and personalized approach to enhancing overall health and well-being for our patients. This integrative approach allows us to better understand and optimize everyone's health needs.

Chapter Nine

Change Your Routine, Improve Your Reality

Imagine a beautiful vision of a world where drugs are not necessary and individuals can enjoy a long and healthy life filled with vitality and laughter.

While it may not be possible to eliminate the need for drugs in some medical conditions, we can move closer to this goal. By educating people about the importance of healthy lifestyle choices, investing in research to understand the root causes of diseases, increasing access to preventive healthcare services, and supporting policies that promote health, we can prevent many chronic diseases from developing in the first place. These steps can help us prioritize the primary prevention of diseases and promote health and well-being for all.

I firmly believe that we are the agents of change and transformation of our lives, and we hold the power to materialize the very realities we envision as our dreams. The first step is to embrace accountability for our well-being. To empower ourselves, we must embark on a journey of lifestyle changes, making conscious and wise choices, and wholeheartedly commit to them for the long term.

My statement finds strong support in the realm of solid scientific evidence, particularly within the emerging field of *epigenetics*. This branch of medicine delves into the intricate mechanisms by which genes are activated and deactivated throughout our lifetime, influenced by cellular signaling processes. Epigenetic code reflects a gene's *phenotype* or the interactions of the genome (DNA) with its environment.

Our bodies constantly adapt to the changing environment. Its impact on the living conditions of each person has the power of shutting down some genes in our DNA while activating others to adapt. This is how humans have managed to survive and evolve for thousands of years.

The development of a disease can be related to the expression or activation of the wrong genes. This process is controlled and determined by our lifestyle choices, including diet, activity, and exercise, and our exposure to toxins, chemicals, and radiation.

We are the masters of our destiny; therefore, we have some degree of control over which genes we select during our lives. Our goals should be to select the good genes that can prevent diseases, inflammation, and cancer and to suppress the bad ones that are making the body vulnerable.

Once again, the new science of epigenetics introduces the concept that there is a clear correlation between nutrition, environment, and our genetic makeup. This delicate balance is always changing, and it could lead to a good outcome or a bad one: the choice is for us to make.

When the cells in our body replicate to make new cells, changes are made at the level of the DNA. Even small changes at this crucial moment can have a great impact on the expression of new genes. The body is constantly changing according to the influences coming from our environment.

The choices we make concerning our diet, supplements, lifestyle, and even our mood have a profound impact on the selection and expression of our genes. Within our DNA, we carry a diverse array of both beneficial and potentially unfavorable genes. An external factor, such as a virus, can interact with our DNA changing the program.

An illustrative instance of this interplay occurs when we contract a viral infection, like the highly oncogenic strain of the common human papillomavirus (HPV), which can induce detrimental alterations in the activity of our genes. Once the virus penetrates the cells, it gives new directions, forcing the cell to produce the oncoproteins mentioned previously, E6 and E7.

Both proteins work together in synchrony, and they are responsible for extending the life of the infected cells. Extending the life of the cells will allow the virus to create thousands of copies of itself over time while strengthening its ability to damage the host DNA, creating precancerous and cancerous lesions in the tissue affected. This is a typical example of how an external factor related to the environment can create changes that can lead to the development of cancer.

A change in our diet and lifestyle can seriously influence our DNA by turning off and on genes responsible for the expression of diseases in the body. Some genes are, for example, in charge of our metabolic rate, weight gain or weight loss, and ability to burn fat and produce muscles.

Diet and exercise can exert a beneficial impact on our brain by elevating the levels of *endorphins* and regulating the production of neurotransmitters like dopamine and serotonin. These effects contribute to enhancing our mood, fostering a more optimistic outlook on life, and reducing the prevalence of anxiety and depression, which often afflict our society.

Selecting good nutrients for our brain can decrease the risk of degenerative diseases such as Alzheimer's, for instance, while improving intellectual ability and functioning. A diet rich in fish and omega-3 fatty acids has the effect of decreasing the genetic expression of cytokines such IL-6 and TNF-alpha, which represent the chemical mediators responsible for producing inflammation in the body.

A down-regulation in the production of cytokines will also have a beneficial effect on the activity of our immune system.

THE MICROBIOME

The *microbiome* is the sum of the bacteria and other microorganisms that colonize the body.

Gut Microbiome

Chronic inflammatory changes in the body are responsible for the most common ailments that affect modern society, and the process starts invariably in the gut.

Establishing a healthy flora in the gut has proven essential to maintaining good health. Much of your immune system's health is influenced by the health of the intestines. Both *good* and *bad* flora colonize the gut. If there is no balance, or if there is a profound majority of *bad* flora, it will affect the immune response.

The presence of "good germs" such as bifidobacteria or lactobacilli strengthens the immune system, produces important nutrients, and gets rid of waste while protecting the integrity of the intestinal tract lining from harmful microorganisms that are ingested with food or drinks.

Maintaining a diverse and advantageous array of gut bacteria facilitates optimal digestive function and improves the absorption of essential nutrients like the B-complex vitamins and vitamin K. These nutrients play crucial roles in significant metabolic processes and cardiovascular health, while also safeguarding the integrity of the blood vessels.

By fostering an alkaline environment in the intestines, beneficial bacteria elevate the pH level, thereby enhancing the body's capacity to eliminate toxins and reducing inflammation throughout our system. The presence of these powerful allies in your digestive system heightens the production of neuro-hormones that positively influence mood, personality, and emotions. This, in turn, ensures healthy brain function and enhances social interactions while promoting overall well-being.

On the other hand, the presence of harmful bacteria in the gastrointestinal tract can be responsible for damaging the lining.

1. **Gluten and the Intestinal Lining**

   a. **Gluten Structure and Digestion:**

   - **Gluten** is a composite of storage proteins found in wheat and related grains like barley and rye. The primary components are **gliadin** and **glutenin**.

   - In individuals with celiac disease or gluten sensitivity, the immune system reacts abnormally to these proteins.

   b. **Autoimmune Response in Celiac Disease:**

   - **Celiac Disease** is an autoimmune disorder where ingestion of gluten triggers an immune response that damages the small intestine.

   - **Immune Mechanism**: When gluten peptides cross the intestinal barrier, they are modified by the enzyme **tissue transglutaminase (tTG)**. This modification makes them more immunogenic, prompting the immune system to attack not only the gluten peptides but also the intestinal lining itself.

2. **Damage to the Intestinal Lining**

   a. **Villous Atrophy:**

- The small intestine is lined with finger-like projections called **villi,** which increase the surface area for nutrient absorption.

- Chronic inflammation from the immune response leads to **villous atrophy,** where these villi become flattened and blunted.

b. Crypt Hyperplasia:

- Alongside villous atrophy, the crypts—glandular structures between villi—can become hyperplastic, increasing in depth as the body attempts to regenerate the damaged epithelium.

3. Consequences of a Compromised Intestinal Barrier

a. Impaired Nutrient Absorption:

- **Nutrient Malabsorption**: Flattened villi reduce the surface area available for absorbing essential nutrients such as vitamins (e.g., B12, D), minerals (e.g., iron, calcium), fats, and proteins.

- **Symptoms**: This can lead to deficiencies, causing anemia, osteoporosis, fatigue, and other systemic issues.

b. Increased Intestinal Permeability ("Leaky Gut"):

- The integrity of the intestinal barrier is maintained by **tight junctions** between epithelial cells. Inflammation and damage disrupt these junctions, increasing permeability.

- **Entry of Toxins and Pathogens**: A leaky gut allows **toxins, pathogenic bacteria, viruses,** and **parasites** to translocate from the gut lumen into the bloodstream and other tissues.

4. **Systemic Implications of Barrier Dysfunction**

   a. **Immune System Activation:**

- The presence of foreign substances in the bloodstream can trigger a chronic immune response, leading to systemic inflammation.

- This systemic inflammation is associated with various autoimmune conditions and may exacerbate existing health issues.

   b. **Exposure to Toxins and Pathogens:**

- **Toxins**: Environmental and dietary toxins that normally would be restricted by the intestinal barrier can enter circulation, potentially affecting organs and contributing to diseases.

- **Pathogens**: There is an increased risk of infections from bacteria, viruses, and parasites that can gain easier access to the body's internal systems.

   c. **Microbiome Imbalance:**

- Damage to the intestinal lining can disrupt the balance of the **gut microbiota**, promoting the growth of harmful bacteria and reducing beneficial microbial populations.

- **Dysbiosis** can further impair immune function and nutrient metabolism.

5. Long-Term Health Consequences

a. Osteoporosis:

- Malabsorption of calcium and vitamin D can lead to weakened bones and increased risk of fractures.

b. Neurological Issues:

- Deficiencies in B vitamins and other nutrients can result in neurological symptoms such as neuropathy, cognitive disturbances, and mood disorders.

c. Increased Risk of Other Autoimmune Diseases:

- Individuals with celiac disease are at a higher risk of developing other autoimmune conditions like Type 1 diabetes, autoimmune thyroiditis, and dermatitis herpetiformis.

d. Enhanced Susceptibility to Infections:

- A compromised barrier and immune dysregulation can make individuals more susceptible to gastrointestinal infections and systemic illnesses.

6. Enzyme Deficiency and Gluten Processing

a. Role of Enzymes:

- Normally, digestive enzymes break down gluten into smaller peptides. In individuals lacking specific enzymes—such as certain proteases—larger, immunogenic gluten fragments persist.

b. Accumulation of Immunogenic Peptides:

- These larger peptides are more likely to trigger an immune response, exacerbating intestinal damage and systemic inflammation.

7. Management and Mitigation

a. Strict Gluten-Free Diet:

- The primary treatment for celiac disease and non-celiac gluten sensitivity is a strict gluten-free diet, which allows the intestinal lining to heal and restores barrier function over time.

b. Nutritional Support:

- Supplementation with deficient nutrients and monitoring bone density can help manage and prevent long-term complications.

c. Potential Therapies:

- Research is ongoing into enzyme supplements that could help break down gluten in the digestive tract, potentially reducing its immunogenicity.

8. Conclusion

For individuals allergic to gluten or lacking the necessary enzymes to process it, the ingestion of gluten can lead to significant and potentially irreversible damage to the intestinal lining. This damage not only impairs nutrient absorption, leading to a host of nutritional deficiencies, but also compromises the intestinal barrier's ability to protect against harmful substances. The resulting systemic inflammation and increased susceptibility to infections underscore the importance of proper diagnosis and management through dietary modifications and medical interventions.

Other Sensitivities

People can have a sensitivity to other food groups as well, such as nightshades or legumes, and not even be aware of symptoms that arise—they may just feel fatigued or out of sorts.

A damaged gut lining will also allow large molecules and toxins to penetrate our blood circulation and the lymphatic system, triggering the immune system to create an inflammatory response that can increase the risk of obesity, diabetes, and cancer and degenerative diseases of the nervous system, such as dementia, Parkinson's, and Alzheimer's.

Oral Microbiome

The oral microbiome refers to the diverse community of microorganisms that reside in the mouth. It is a complex ecosystem composed of bacteria, viruses, fungi, and other microorganisms. When this ecosystem is in balance, it can contribute positively to various aspects of oral health, digestion, and overall well-being. However, imbalances or disruptions in the oral microbiome can lead to various oral and systemic health issues.

Maintaining a balanced oral microbiome is crucial for overall health and plays a significant role in preventing various diseases, including *hypertension* or high blood pressure.

The oral microbiome affects overall health and its connection to preventing hypertension:

- *Oral Health.* A balanced oral microbiome helps to maintain healthy teeth and gums. Harmful bacteria in the mouth can lead to dental issues such as tooth decay—cavities—and periodontal or gum disease. If left untreated, these oral health problems can contribute to systemic inflammation, which is a risk factor for hypertension and other chronic diseases.

- *Inflammation.* Imbalances in the oral microbiome can trigger inflammation in the mouth and, subsequently, throughout the body. Chronic inflammation is associated with an increased risk of hypertension and other cardiovascular diseases. Bacteria and toxins from the mouth can enter the bloodstream and contribute to inflammation, which may negatively impact blood vessel function and increase blood pressure.

- *Nitric Oxide Production.* A healthy oral microbiome can help to produce nitric oxide, a molecule that plays a key role in regulating blood pressure. Nitric oxide helps blood vessels relax, which improves blood flow and reduces blood pressure. However, certain harmful bacteria in the mouth can interfere with nitric oxide production, potentially contributing to hypertension.

- *Gut Microbiome Interaction.* The oral microbiome is connected to the gut microbiome, which is another essential ecosystem of microorganisms in the digestive system. Disruptions in the oral microbiome can lead to imbalances in the gut microbiome, affecting overall digestion and nutrient absorption. These gut-related issues have been linked to hypertension and other cardiovascular problems.

To maintain a balanced oral microbiome and promote overall health, consider the following practices:

- Brush your teeth at least twice a day and floss daily to remove plaque and food particles that can lead to bacterial growth.

- Visit your dentist regularly for check-ups and cleanings to identify and address any oral health issues promptly.

- Consume a balanced diet rich in fruits and vegetables, while minimizing sugary and processed foods.

- Avoid tobacco and limit alcohol consumption.

- Consider using alcohol-free mouthwash or oral hygiene products that do not disrupt the natural flora balance.

- Stay hydrated, as saliva plays a critical role in maintaining a balanced oral microbiome.

- Manage stress, as it can impact both oral and overall health.

By promoting a healthy oral microbiome, you can contribute to your overall well-being and potentially reduce the risk of hypertension and other systemic diseases. Remember that oral health is an integral part of maintaining a healthy body.

Pro- and Prebiotics

The intake of pro- and prebiotics in your diet will have the effect of improving the quality and the selection of the bacterial flora.

Taking probiotics will help, but it is also essential to provide good bacteria with enough nutrients to survive and thrive in the gut.

Our diet must be supported by introducing enough fiber, ideally twenty to thirty grams daily by means of complex carbohydrates, such as brown rice and sweet potatoes.

Plenty of green leafy vegetables and some fruits are important because they add nutritional value while boosting the level of alkalinity of our system.

1. **The Protective Gut Lining**

    •   **Function**: The lining of your gut acts as a barrier, controlling what gets absorbed into your bloodstream. It allows essential nutrients to pass through while keeping harmful substances out.

    •   **Components**: This barrier consists of tightly packed cells and protective mucus that prevent unwanted particles like toxins, harmful chemicals, bad bacteria, and parasites from entering your body.

2. **Compromised Gut Barrier**

    •   **What Happens**: When the gut lining is damaged—due to factors like gluten intolerance, chronic inflammation, infections, or poor diet—it becomes "leaky." This condition is often referred to as **"leaky gut syndrome."**

    •   **Consequences of a Leaky Gut:**

        •   **Toxin Absorption**: Harmful substances that are normally blocked can pass through the gut lining into the bloodstream.

        •   **Immune System Activation**: The body recognizes these unwanted particles as threats, triggering an immune response.

3. **The Inflammatory Response**

    •   **Purpose**: Inflammation is the body's natural way of fighting off harmful substances. It aims to eliminate toxins, pathogens, and other contaminants that have entered the bloodstream.

- **Short-Term vs. Long-Term:**

  - **Short-Term Inflammation**: This helps heal injuries and fight infections.

  - **Chronic Inflammation**: When inflammation persists over a long period, it can start causing more harm than good.

4. **Chronic Inflammation and Health Risks**

Prolonged inflammation due to a compromised gut barrier can contribute to various serious health issues:

- **Obesity**

  - **How**: Chronic inflammation can disrupt metabolism and hormone regulation, leading to weight gain and difficulty losing weight.

- **Diabetes**

  - **How**: Inflammation can impair insulin signaling, increasing insulin resistance and the risk of developing type 2 diabetes.

- **Cancer**

  - **How**: Ongoing inflammation can cause DNA damage and promote an environment that supports cancer cell growth.

- **Degenerative Nervous System Diseases**

  - **Dementia, Parkinson's, Alzheimer's**

    - **How**: Inflammatory molecules can cross into the brain, leading to neuronal damage, impaired cognitive functions, and the progression of neurodegenerative diseases.

5. **Impact on the Immune System**

   - **Overactive Immune Response**: Chronic exposure to harmful substances keeps the immune system in a constant state of activation, which can weaken its ability to respond effectively to actual threats.

   - **Autoimmune Diseases**: The immune system may start attacking the body's own tissues, mistaking them for harmful invaders, leading to conditions like rheumatoid arthritis or lupus.

6. **Summary of the Chain Reaction**

   - **Gut Lining Damage**: Happens due to factors like gluten intolerance, enzyme deficiency, or poor diet.

   - **Leaky Gut**: Allows toxins, harmful chemicals, bad bacteria, and parasites to enter the bloodstream.

   - **Immune Response**: Initiates inflammation to eliminate these contaminants from the body.

   - **Chronic Inflammation**: Leads to systemic issues when prolonged.

   - **Health Risks**: Increases the likelihood of obesity, diabetes, cancer, and neurodegenerative diseases.

7. **Mitigating the Risks**

   - **Maintain Gut Health**

     - **Balanced Diet**: Eat foods rich in fiber, probiotics, and anti-inflammatory ingredients.

- **Avoid Triggers**: Gluten is contraindicated for those with sensitivities or intolerances.

- **Manage Inflammation**

  - **Lifestyle Changes**: Regular exercise, adequate sleep, and stress management support the body.

  - **Medical Intervention**: Consult healthcare providers for appropriate treatments and supplements.

- **Regular Check-Ups**

  - **Monitoring Health**: Regular screenings can help detect and address issues early before they develop into more serious conditions.

Conclusion

A healthy gut lining is crucial for preventing harmful substances from entering your bloodstream and triggering chronic inflammation.

Maintaining gut integrity through proper diet, lifestyle, and medical care can significantly reduce the risk of developing a range of serious health issues related to chronic inflammation.

Aloe Vera

In his 2022 edition book titled *HPV, Pap Smears, Cervical Dysplasia, and Warts*, C. W. Willington discusses several reports and testimonials highlighting the significance of incorporating aloe-vera-derived supplements, specifically a product known as Beta-mannan, to support the body in its efforts to clear the virus.

Aloe vera is a succulent plant that has been used for various medicinal and cosmetic purposes for centuries. While it's often praised for its potential health benefits, scientific research of the specific effects of aloe vera on the immune system is limited and often inconclusive.

Aloe vera does contain various bioactive compounds—including vitamins, minerals, enzymes, polysaccharides, and others—that could potentially have immune-modulating properties. Some studies suggest that these compounds might have anti-inflammatory and antioxidant effects, which could indirectly support immune system function by reducing oxidative stress and inflammation. (Kumar, et al. 2019)

However, more research is needed to fully understand these potential effects and their impact on the immune system.

No peer-reviewed studies are available to substantiate the claimed effectiveness of the supplement. On the other hand, I have found in medical literature a study done in rats that shows a clear relationship between extract from aloe vera plant intake and onset of cancer in the gastrointestinal tract. (Boudreau, et al. 2013)

These studies prompt caution when considering a systemic intake of supplements extracted from this plant.

INFLAMMATION'S ADVERSE EFFECT ON YOUR HEALTH

Inflammation is a natural immune response triggered by the body to protect itself from harmful stimuli, such as pathogens, injuries, or irritants. It is a vital defense mechanism that helps the body repair damaged tissues, fight infections, and maintain overall homeostasis.

The process of inflammation involves a complex interplay of cells, chemicals, and molecular signals. When the body detects an injury or an invasion of pathogens, immune cells release signaling molecules like *cytokines* and *chemokines*. These molecules attract other immune cells to the affected area, leading to an influx of white blood cells and immune mediators.

The inflammatory process can damage tissues and organs, disrupt normal cellular functions, and create an environment conducive to disease development. Many common diseases—including cardiovascular diseases, diabetes, arthritis, neurodegenerative disorders, and certain cancers—have been linked to chronic inflammation.

In acute inflammation, this response is short-lived and helps the body heal. However, chronic inflammation is a different story. It occurs when the inflammatory response persists over a prolonged period, potentially lasting for months or even years. Chronic inflammation can arise due to various factors, including persistent infections, exposure to toxins, autoimmune disorders, or lifestyle factors such as poor diet, lack of exercise, and stress.

Here are some key aspects of inflammation's role in specific health conditions:

- *Cancer.* Chronic inflammation has been linked to an increased risk of cancer development and progression. It can promote the growth and spread of cancer cells, as well as hinder the body's ability to recognize and eliminate abnormal cells.

- *Aging.* Chronic inflammation has been proposed as one of the contributors to the aging process. Over time, the persistent presence of inflammatory molecules can damage tissues and cellular structures, leading to age-related decline and dysfunction.

- *Weight gain and obesity.* Chronic low-grade inflammation in fat tissue is associated with obesity and metabolic disorders. *Adipose tissue*, or fat cells, produce pro-inflammatory molecules, contributing to insulin resistance and other obesity-related complications.

- *Diabetes.* Inflammation can impair the function of insulin-producing cells in the pancreas and reduce the body's sensitivity to insulin, leading to diabetes or worsening glycemic control in individuals with existing diabetes.

- *Degenerative brain diseases (Alzheimer's, dementia).* Chronic inflammation in the brain can damage nerve cells and disrupt normal brain function. In conditions like Alzheimer's and dementia, the presence of inflammatory markers has been observed in affected brain regions.

While inflammation plays a significant role in these conditions, it is not the sole cause. These conditions are often multifactorial involving a combination of genetic, environmental, and lifestyle factors.

Managing inflammation is a crucial aspect of maintaining overall health. A balanced diet, regular exercise, stress management, and avoiding tobacco and excessive alcohol use can all help reduce the risk of chronic inflammation. Medical professionals may also prescribe anti-inflammatory medications in certain situations. However, the underlying causes of inflammation should always be addressed to achieve long-term health benefits.

A *wrong diet*—one rich in processed food, meat, eggs, and farm-raised fish derived from livestock fed a non-natural diet such as grains—is the number one cause of inflammation in our bodies.

Deli meat, processed food, and some canned goods are widely available and often more affordable grocery options, but they can also be considered among the most harmful choices for our health. These foods are commonly associated with several adverse health effects, making them *deadly* in terms of their potential impact on our well-being.

Here's a more comprehensive explanation:

- *Deli meat.* Deli meats, such as ham, salami, sausages, and bacon, are typically high in sodium, saturated fats, and preservatives. Regular consumption of processed meats has been linked to an increased risk of heart disease, stroke, and certain types of cancer, particularly colorectal cancer. Additionally, the nitrites and nitrates used as preservatives in deli meat can form harmful compounds when metabolized in the body.

- *Processed food.* Processed foods, including ready-to-eat meals, snacks, and sugary treats, often contain high levels of added sugars, sodium, unhealthy fats, and artificial additives. Regularly consuming processed foods is associated with a higher risk of obesity, type 2 diabetes, hypertension, and other chronic diseases. These foods are often calorie-dense and nutrient-poor, leading to imbalanced diets and potential nutritional deficiencies.

- *Canned goods.* While canned goods like vegetables, fruits, and soups offer convenience and longer shelf life, some concerns arise from the canning process. Many canned products contain added sugars, sodium, and preservatives to enhance flavor and prolong shelf life. The lining of some cans also contains bisphenol A (BPA), a chemical that may leach into the food and has been associated with adverse health effects, including hormonal disruption.

Although these affordable options may be more convenient and readily available, it is essential to recognize their potential health risks. It is advisable to prioritize whole, fresh foods, such as fruits, vegetables, and lean proteins, which offer more significant nutritional benefits and contribute to better long-term health outcomes. While they may require longer preparation, planning, and money, the investment in a healthier diet can lead to significant improvements in overall health and well-being.

Mechanism by Which the Body Deals With Toxic Overload:

The body has various mechanisms to deal with toxins and chemicals that enter the system through exposure to the environment or dietary sources, among them:

Storage. In some cases, the body may store these toxic substances to prevent immediate harm to critical organs or systems. Two common storage locations for toxins are adipose tissue (fat cells) and bones.

Fat cells can act as a repository for fat-soluble toxins, while bones can store heavy metals like lead and cadmium. By subtracting these substances from the bloodstream, the body aims to minimize their immediate impact on health. Organs like fat and bones have a lower blood supply compared to other vital organs like the heart, liver, and kidneys. The reduced blood flow to these storage sites helps limit the circulation of stored toxins and their potential to cause harm. The downside, however, is that these stored toxins can persist in the body for long periods, potentially causing health issues if not addressed.

Water retention. By retaining more water, the body attempts to dilute the concentration of toxins and chemicals in the bloodstream, reducing their immediate impact on sensitive organs and tissues. In some cases, chronic water retention could indeed be an indicator of high toxin levels in the body. However, it's essential to recognize that water retention can also be caused by various other factors, such as hormonal imbalances, certain medications, heart and kidney conditions, and dietary factors—e.g., excessive sodium intake. Therefore, the presence of water retention alone may not be enough to confirm high toxicity levels; it should be assessed in conjunction with other symptoms and health markers.

Rapid weight gain and inflammation. Chronic inflammation is the body's response to various stimuli, such as infection, injury, or exposure to toxins. Inflammatory processes can lead to fluid retention, which contributes to weight gain. Remember that water is heavier than fat. However, it's crucial to differentiate between healthy weight gain—e.g., muscle gain through exercise—and unhealthy weight gain caused by inflammation and chronic health issues.

Overall, the body employs several protective mechanisms to deal with toxins and chemicals. Understanding these processes can highlight the importance of minimizing exposure to harmful substances and adopting a healthy lifestyle that includes a balanced diet, regular exercise, and adequate hydration. If you suspect a high toxic burden, consult with a healthcare professional and undergo appropriate testing to identify and address any underlying health issues.

Gastrointestinal Health

Many patients in my daily medical practice frequently express a common set of complaints related to their gastrointestinal health. They often report feeling bloated, experiencing chronic constipation, and finding it difficult to digest their food properly. Additionally, they frequently complain about feeling tired and sluggish. These symptoms are of significant concern to them and impact on their overall well-being.

Some of them will even go through highly invasive medical procedures such as colonoscopies, upper GI endoscopies, CT scans, and ultrasound to come up with no identified cause for their symptoms. It can be a long, expensive, and frustrating path that leads nowhere.

A common reason for digestive trouble is often inflammatory changes occurring at the level of the lining of the gut. This inflammatory process could be difficult to identify early in the process even with sophisticated tests such as endoscopy or colonoscopy.

Tight junctions among the cells that line our gut are called *gap junctions*. These gap junctions regulate the absorption of nutrients and water from the food ingested into the blood supply. A disruption of the intestinal lining will alter the ability of the gut to exercise its function, and it will allow large molecules like gluten, proteins, bacteria, and toxins to penetrate the blood circulation, causing further damage and more inflammation. This condition, called *leaky gut syndrome*, is quite common these days. (Camilleri 2019, 2021; Usuda, et al. 2021)

Restoring the normal function of the gut and rebalancing the gut microbiota can have significant positive impacts on both digestive health and overall well-being.

The following factors can help shift gut health:

- *Dietary Changes.* A well-balanced and nutritious diet is crucial for gut health. Include a variety of fruits, vegetables, whole grains, lean proteins, and healthy fats to provide essential nutrients and support the gut's healing process. Avoid processed foods, excessive sugar, and unhealthy fats.

- *Prebiotics and Probiotics. Prebiotics* are nondigestible fibers that serve as food for beneficial gut bacteria. They can be found in foods like bananas, garlic, onions, asparagus, and whole grains. *Probiotics* are live beneficial bacteria found in certain foods— e.g., yogurt, kefir, sauerkraut—or supplements. Consuming both prebiotic- and probiotic-rich foods helps foster a balanced gut microbiome.

- *Avoiding Triggers.* Identifying and avoiding foods that worsen gut symptoms is essential. Common triggers include spicy foods, caffeine, alcohol, and certain food intolerances. A food diary may help patients pinpoint problematic foods.

- *Special Diets for Gut Healing.* There are specific diets that focus on gut healing, such as the Low FODMAP Diet, which temporarily restricts certain fermentable carbohydrates to reduce gut symptoms. Another example is the Specific Carbohydrate Diet (SCD), which aims to promote gut healing by avoiding complex carbohydrates and processed foods.

- *Hydration.* Staying well-hydrated is important for gut health. Drinking enough water supports digestive function and helps prevent constipation.

- *Stress management.* Chronic stress can negatively impact gut health. Managing stress through relaxation techniques, exercise, and mindfulness can be beneficial.

- *Exercise.* Regular physical activity like walking supports overall health, including gut function. Exercise can help alleviate constipation and promote healthy bowel movements.

- *Adequate Sleep.* Sleep is vital for overall health and can also influence gut health. Establish good sleep habits to support your digestive system.

- *Digestive enzymes.* These can play a crucial role in supporting digestion and alleviating some of the common complaints of feeling bloated, having difficulty digesting food, and feeling sluggish. These enzymes are naturally produced by the body, and their primary function is to break down complex nutrients into smaller, more easily absorbable molecules.

They help in several ways:

- *Improved Nutrient Absorption.* Enzymes aid in the breakdown of carbohydrates, proteins, and fats present in the diet. By breaking down these complex molecules into smaller units— e.g., sugars, amino acids, fatty acids—the body can efficiently absorb and utilize the nutrients. This can be especially beneficial for individuals who may have deficiencies due to poor nutrient absorption.

- *Reduced Bloating and Gas.* When food is not adequately broken down during digestion, it can lead to the fermentation of undigested carbohydrates in the gut by bacteria, resulting in bloating and gas. Digestive enzymes can help prevent this by enhancing the digestion process.

- *Alleviation of Digestive Discomfort.* For individuals who experience discomfort after meals, such as heaviness or indigestion, taking digestive enzymes with their meals can help ease the burden on the digestive system and reduce these discomforts.

- *Support for Enzyme Deficiencies.* Some people may have conditions that lead to enzyme deficiencies, such as pancreatic insufficiency. Other patients might miss their gallbladder through surgical intervention. The gallbladder plays an important role in the digestive process because it stores bile, which is essential for the digestion of fat and disposal of toxins and metabolic waste. The organ responds by releasing bile when the digestive tract needs it the most. In such cases, supplementing with the specific missing enzymes can be beneficial for digestion and nutrient absorption.

- *Enhanced Gut Health.* By promoting better digestion and reducing the presence of undigested food in the gut, digestive enzymes can help maintain a healthier gut environment and support a balanced gut microbiome.

- *Support During Aging.* As we age, the body's production of digestive enzymes may decrease, leading to potential digestive issues. Supplementing enzymes can help address this age-related decline.

While digestive enzyme supplements can be helpful for some individuals, they may not be necessary or suitable for everyone. Before starting any supplements, patients should consult with a healthcare professional, such as a registered dietitian or gastroenterologist, to tailor a plan that suits the patient's specific needs and health conditions.

Additionally, addressing underlying dietary and lifestyle factors, such as eating a balanced diet, managing stress, and staying physically active, should remain foundational in improving gut health and digestion. Digestive enzymes can be a helpful addition to a comprehensive approach to gut health, but they are not a replacement for a healthy lifestyle and a well-balanced diet.

Remember, the gut is a complex and interconnected system, so addressing gut health can have far-reaching effects on general health and vitality. By taking a holistic approach and making informed choices, patients can often experience notable improvements in their well-being.

THE ROLE OF REGENERATIVE MEDICINE

Regenerative medicine recognizes that chronic inflammation in the body can play a significant role in the development and progression of numerous prevalent diseases. Inflammation is a natural immune response that helps the body fight infections and heal injuries. However, when inflammation becomes chronic or dysregulated, it can lead to tissue damage and cellular dysfunction and contribute to the pathogenesis of various conditions.

Understanding Regenerative Medicine

Regenerative medicine is a groundbreaking and swiftly progressing branch of healthcare that focuses on restoring the function of damaged tissues and organs by leveraging the body's inherent healing mechanisms. Unlike traditional medicine, which often aims to manage symptoms or halt disease progression, regenerative medicine seeks to repair or replace the underlying damaged structures, offering the potential for more permanent and effective solutions.

Harnessing the Body's Natural Healing Abilities

At the core of regenerative medicine is the principle of utilizing the body's own capacity to heal itself. This involves stimulating the natural processes that repair tissues, such as:

- **Stem Cell Therapy**: Stem cells have the unique ability to differentiate into various cell types. By introducing stem cells into damaged areas, regenerative medicine can encourage the formation of new, healthy cells to replace those that are diseased or injured.

- **Growth Factors, Exosomes and Cytokines**: These are proteins and messengers that play crucial roles in cell signaling, guiding the growth, differentiation, and survival of cells. By manipulating these factors, scientists can direct the regeneration process more precisely.

- **Tissue Engineering**: This involves creating biological substitutes that can restore, maintain, or improve tissue function. Combining scaffolds—structures that support cell growth—with cells and biologically active molecules can lead to the formation of new tissue.

Personalized Approach to Medicine

Regenerative medicine emphasizes a personalized strategy, recognizing that each patient is unique in terms of their genetic makeup, lifestyle, environment, and overall health. This individualized approach involves:

- **Genetic Profiling**: Understanding a patient's genetic predisposition helps tailor treatments that are more effective and reduce the risk of adverse reactions.

- **Environmental Interactions**: Considering how a patient's environment—such as exposure to toxins, lifestyle choices, and social factors—affects their health allows for more comprehensive treatment plans.

- **Customized Therapies**: Treatments are designed to align with the specific needs and conditions of each patient, ensuring that the regenerative processes are optimized for their unique situation.

Holistic Treatment of the Body as an Integrated System

Regenerative medicine doesn't just focus on isolated parts of the body; it treats the entire body as an interconnected system. This holistic perspective means:

- **Inter-Organ Communication**: Recognizing that organs and tissues communicate through complex signaling networks, regenerative medicine aims to restore balance and harmony across the entire system. For example, improving liver function can have positive effects on overall metabolism and energy levels.

- **Systemic Health Improvement**: By addressing the root causes of ailments rather than just the symptoms, regenerative treatments can lead to overall health improvements. For instance, regenerating damaged heart tissue not only improves cardiac function but also enhances circulation and reduces strain on other organs.

- **Symphony of Healing**: Just as different sections of an orchestra work together to create harmonious music, various regenerative processes collaborate to restore health. This coordinated effort ensures that healing is comprehensive and sustained.

Identifying Root Causes and Developing Innovative Methods

A key strength of regenerative medicine is its focus on understanding and addressing the underlying causes of diseases and injuries. This involves:

- **Advanced Diagnostics**: Utilize cutting-edge imaging and molecular diagnostics to pinpoint the exact sources of damage or dysfunction.

- **Mechanistic Insights**: Gain a deep understanding of the biological mechanisms that lead to tissue damage, such as inflammation, cellular senescence, or genetic mutations.

- **Innovative Therapies**: Develop new treatment modalities that target these mechanisms directly. For example, gene editing technologies can correct genetic defects that cause certain diseases, while bioactive materials can provide scaffolding for tissue regeneration.

Promoting Tissue Growth and Repair

Regenerative medicine employs various strategies to encourage the growth and repair of tissues, ensuring that the body can recover effectively:

- **Biomaterials**: These are engineered substances that can support the growth of new tissues by providing a scaffold for cells to attach and proliferate.

- **Cell-Based Therapies**: Introducing specific cell types, such as mesenchymal stem cells, to damaged areas can facilitate the regeneration of tissues like bone, cartilage, and muscle.

- **3D Bioprinting**: This technology allows for the precise layering of cells and biomaterials to create complex tissue structures, paving the way for the regeneration of entire organs in the future.

Enhancing Overall Health and Well-Being

The individualized and holistic nature of regenerative medicine leads to numerous benefits that extend beyond treating specific ailments:

- **Improved Quality of Life**: By effectively addressing the root causes of health issues, patients experience better long-term outcomes and enhanced daily functioning.

- **Reduced Dependency on Medications**: Successful regenerative treatments can decrease the need for ongoing pharmaceutical interventions, minimizing potential side effects and healthcare costs.

- **Preventative Health**: Understanding and treating underlying health vulnerabilities can prevent the onset of more serious conditions, promoting longevity and sustained well-being.

Real-World Applications and Future Prospects

Regenerative medicine is already making significant impacts in various areas:

- **Orthopedics**: Regenerates cartilage in joints to treat osteoarthritis, reducing the need for joint replacement surgeries.

- **Cardiology**: Repairs heart tissue after myocardial infarctions (heart attacks) to improve cardiac function and reduce the risk of heart failure.

- **Neurology**: Explores treatments for neurodegenerative diseases like Parkinson's and Alzheimer's by regenerating damaged neurons.

Looking ahead, the future of regenerative medicine holds immense promise:

- **Organ Regeneration**: Advances in stem cell research and tissue engineering may one day enable the regeneration of entire organs, alleviating transplant shortages and eliminating the need for immunosuppressive drugs.

- **Personalized Regenerative Therapies**: As our understanding of individual genetic and molecular profiles deepens, treatments will become even more tailored, increasing their effectiveness and safety.

- **Integration with Other Technologies**: Combining regenerative medicine with technologies like artificial intelligence and nanotechnology could lead to unprecedented advancements in healthcare.

Conclusion

Regenerative medicine represents a paradigm shift in how we approach health and healing. By embracing a personalized and holistic framework, it not only targets the specific causes of diseases and injuries but also fosters a harmonious restoration of the body's entire system. This innovative field holds the potential to revolutionize medical treatments, offering more effective and enduring solutions that significantly enhance overall health and quality of life.

CHAPTER TEN

THE PURSUIT OF WELLNESS
THROUGH LIFESTYLE CHOICES

In a world characterized by uncertainty, inequality, and swift changes, maintaining our faith and hope can become challenging.

We must hold on to those core values that we believe in and can give real meaning to our lives. Recognizing the paramount importance of safeguarding our physical well-being and the soundness of our bodies serves as the cornerstone for leading a productive life, forming a solid foundation for our families, and establishing the bedrock of a robust and thriving community infrastructure.

A famous Latin saying derived from Greek culture expresses the concept of "Mens sana in corpore sano," which translates to: "a healthy mind resides in a healthy body."

I support this concept because I have seen and experienced it directly and indirectly through my professional life.

While we have myriad choices of healing modalities, practitioners, and treatments or medicines available to us, there are also many ways in which we create and sustain wellness that are simply based in how we live each day. These lifestyle choices are within our grasp and do not require any prescription. In the end, it's up to us to choose whether we pursue a path of health or continue down the road of illness.

NUTRITION

We need to stay healthy by providing our body with nutritious food, rich in vitamins, proteins, enzymes, and antioxidants that are so important in keeping our system running efficiently. Making mindful and selective choices while grocery shopping is essential for supporting our nutritional needs and overall health. Before adding any food item to the cart, we should ask ourselves whether each item will benefit our body's nutritional requirements or potentially harm our well-being. By adopting this approach, we can prioritize wholesome foods that nourish our bodies and discard junk food that can have the opposite effect.

Being conscious of our food choices empowers us to take control of our diet and make decisions that promote vitality and long-term well-being. We need to avoid the intake of food with preservatives, excessive salt, heavy metals, dyes, GMOs, hydrocarbons, high fructose corn syrup, and refined sugar. Please read the labels!

A healthy and balanced diet has a positive effect not only on the body but also on the mind, boosting our mood and increasing our ability to focus and be productive. Additionally, it decreases the risk of inflammatory and degenerative disorders that can severely affect the brain and predispose us to diseases like Alzheimer's, dementia, and autoimmune neurological disorders.

In addition to good nourishment, several other lifestyle factors come into play, which we explore in depth in this chapter.

Restorative sleep improves our physical, emotional, and intellectual functioning.

Daily physical exercise and meditation sharpen our mental skills and allow us to exercise better control over our minds.

The ability to clear any thoughts from our mind is an important learning process that benefits us immensely to control the stress and anxiety that seem to be common in modern society.

To keep our stress level under control, we need to find a happy, safe place inside ourselves and shield our minds from harmful negative emotions, toxic information, and harsh environments. A consistent practice of yoga and meditation can help us establish an intimate conversation with the deeper and more authentic parts of ourselves.

We need to find time and space to cultivate ourselves; fill ourselves first; make ourselves happy and fulfilled with meaningful activities such as physical exercise, reading, listening to music, dancing, and being involved with social activities and volunteer work; and dedicate enough time to friends and family.

HAPPINESS

Humans ultimately share the same goal: the pursuit of happiness. Happiness is not something you can buy or something other people can give to you.

Do not depend on other people to find happiness.

Happiness is not a choice but can be a goal. We can certainly set up the best conditions to be happy by creating a work-life balance or by reframing how we see reality for positivity; in other words, we can research a different perspective of the reality we live in that carries a more positive interpretation.

Keeping a happiness score and making happiness a daily goal can be transformative for our well-being and overall life satisfaction.

Here are some tips to accomplish that:

- *Measuring happiness.* Keeping a happiness score involves regularly evaluating and reflecting on your emotional state and overall contentment.

  It could be as simple as rating your daily happiness on a scale from 1 to 10 or maintaining a journal in which you record your positive experiences and moments of joy. By actively monitoring your happiness, you become more aware of the factors that influence it.

- *Daily goal of happiness.* Making happiness a daily goal shifts your focus toward actively seeking and cultivating moments of joy and contentment. Instead of waiting for external circumstances to bring you happiness, you take responsibility for your own well-being and actively engage in activities and practices that nourish your happiness.

- *Universal pursuit of happiness.* The pursuit of happiness is a fundamental and shared aspiration among humans. Irrespective of cultural backgrounds, ethnicities, or beliefs, we all seek happiness and fulfillment in our lives. Recognizing this common goal can foster a sense of unity and understanding among people.

- *Intrinsic nature of happiness.* True happiness is not reliant on material possessions nor external validation from others. While external factors can contribute to temporary happiness, lasting and meaningful happiness comes from within. It arises from the way you perceive yourself and respond to the world around you.

- *Empowerment in choosing happiness.* By focusing on the positive aspects of your life, you will empower yourself to take charge of your emotions and actions. You can shape your mindset towards a more positive attitude and behavior regardless of external circumstances.

- *Gratitude and positive mindset.* Cultivating gratitude and maintaining a positive mindset are powerful ways to enhance your happiness. By focusing on the positive aspects of your life and acknowledging what you are grateful for, you can shift your perspective toward a more optimistic and contented outlook. People who have great appreciation for who they are and exude love for themselves are the most accomplished people on the planet. Experiencing gratitude for who you are and your unique skills and abilities can help you to overcome difficulties.

- *Self-care and well-being.* Prioritizing self-care, including physical, mental, and emotional well-being, is crucial for nurturing happiness. Engaging in activities that bring you joy, taking time for relaxation and leisure, and fostering meaningful connections with others all contribute to your overall happiness.

- *Balance and authenticity.* Striving for happiness doesn't mean avoiding negative emotions or life's challenges. It's about finding a balance and embracing the full range of human experiences while remaining authentic to yourself and your values.

Boosting your level of happiness could be a very simple and inexpensive process that starts with giving yourself the gift of a smile. A smile is indeed a simple and cost-free way to create positivity within ourselves and others.

Here's why a smile is so powerful:

- *Instant mood booster.* When you smile, your brain releases endorphins, dopamine, and serotonin—the feel-good neurotransmitters. This leads to an immediate improvement in mood, reducing stress and anxiety.

- *Positive attitude.* Smiling can help shift your attitude toward a more positive outlook. It reminds us to focus on the bright side of things and approach challenges with optimism.

- *Infectious happiness.* Smiles are contagious. When you smile at others, it often prompts them to smile back, creating a positive chain reaction and fostering a sense of connection and goodwill.

- *Improved relationships.* Smiling can strengthen interpersonal bonds. It conveys warmth and approachability, making it easier for others to connect with you and feel at ease.

- *Stress reduction.* Smiling can help alleviate the physiological response to stress. It activates the body's relaxation response, promoting a sense of calmness.

- *Enhanced immune system.* Studies suggest the positive emotions associated with smiling can boost the immune system, helping the body better cope with illnesses.

- *Natural beauty.* A smile is one of the most attractive features a person can have. It enhances your facial appearance and makes you more appealing to others.

- *Increased self-confidence.* Smiling can also improve your self-confidence. When you smile, you feel more self-assured and capable, which positively impacts how you interact with others and approach various situations.

- *Eases social interactions.* Smiling can act as a social lubricant, making social interactions more comfortable and enjoyable. It breaks the ice and helps build rapport.

- *Promotes a positive environment.* When you smile in a group setting, you contribute to creating a positive and friendly atmosphere, making the environment more pleasant for everyone.

In conclusion, by actively monitoring your happiness, setting it as a daily goal, and recognizing its intrinsic nature, you empower yourself to lead a happier and more fulfilling life. It's a journey of self-discovery and self-compassion, as you learn to give yourself the gift of happiness each day.

In a world where stress and negativity can often prevail, a simple smile can be a powerful tool to bring light, warmth, and comfort to ourselves and those around us.

It costs nothing but has the potential to enrich our lives and the lives of others in numerous ways. So, let's share the gift of a smile freely and brighten the world with its positive effects.

BREATHING

Another way to create positive changes in your life is to exercise deep breathing.

Deep breathing, also known as *diaphragmatic* or *belly breathing*, is a powerful and accessible tool for bringing happiness, stability, and stress relief into our lives.

The benefits of deep breathing are numerous:

- *Mindfulness and present moment awareness.* Deep breathing encourages you to be fully present in the moment. By focusing on the rhythm of your breath, you anchor your attention to the present and let go of worries about the past or future. This mindfulness practice helps reduce anxiety and enhances your overall sense of well-being.

- *Stress reduction and relaxation.* Deep breathing triggers the body's relaxation response, activating the parasympathetic nervous system. As a result, heart rate and blood pressure decrease, muscle tension eases, and stress hormones, such as cortisol, reduce. This calms the body and mind, promoting a sense of tranquility and stability.

- *Enhanced healing response.* When you breathe deeply, you take in more oxygen, which is essential for your body's healing processes. Oxygen supports cellular function and boosts energy levels, aiding the body's natural ability to repair and restore itself.

- *Reduction of external and internal noise.* Deep breathing allows you to disconnect from the external distractions and noise around you. By focusing inward on your breath, you create a space of calm amid the chaos of the outside world.

- *Quieting the mind.* The practice of deep breathing helps quiet the incessant chatter of the mind. As you concentrate on the rhythm of your breath, you reduce the mental clutter and obsessive, persistent thoughts that can contribute to stress and anxiety.

- *Lowering stress levels.* Deep breathing activates the relaxation response, counteracting the body's stress response. This shift in physiological state helps lower stress levels, making you more resilient to the challenges you encounter.

- *Improved brain function.* By calming the mind and reducing stress, deep breathing can improve cognitive function, focus, and concentration. It allows you to think more clearly and to make better decisions.

- *Coping with emotional distress.* When you practice deep breathing during times of emotional distress, it can help you process your feelings more effectively. It allows you to observe your emotions without being overwhelmed by them, fostering emotional stability.

- *Empowerment in self-regulation.* Deep breathing is a portable and accessible tool that you can use at any time. It empowers you to take control of your emotional and physiological responses, enabling you to navigate life's challenges with greater resilience.

- *Promotion of overall well-being.* Consistent practice of deep breathing can have a cumulative effect on your overall well-being. It becomes a positive habit that supports physical, mental, and emotional health.

Incorporating deep breathing into our daily routine, even for just a few minutes a day, can make a significant difference in our overall happiness and stability. It is a gentle and effective way to nurture a sense of inner peace and balance in our fast-paced and sometimes stressful lives.

EMBRACING POSITIVITY

Regaining control over our lives and embracing each day with positivity and strength are essential for leading fulfilling and meaningful lives.

Here's why these aspects are so crucial:

- *Empowerment.* Feeling that you can regain control of your life empowers you to shape your destiny and make choices that align with your values and goals. It shifts the focus from being a passive recipient of circumstances to being an active participant in creating the life you desire.

- *Resilience.* Embracing each day with positivity and strength fosters resilience. Life can present challenges and setbacks. By maintaining a positive outlook, you develop the mental fortitude to bounce back and overcome obstacles.

- *Improved mental health.* When you embrace positivity and focus on your strengths, it positively impacts your mental well-being. It reduces the prevalence of negative thought patterns, anxiety, and depression, leading to greater emotional stability.

- *Better physical health.* A positive mindset and inner strength can have a direct impact on physical health. Stress reduction, improved sleep, and healthier habits often result from a positive outlook on life.

- *Enhanced relationships.* Positivity and inner strength can lead to healthier and more meaningful relationships. By focusing on empathy, understanding, and communication, you foster a positive environment for your interactions with others.

- *Personal growth.* Regaining control of your life allows you to engage in continuous self-improvement and personal growth. It enables you to identify areas for development and work toward becoming the best versions of yourself.

- *Appreciation of the present.* Embracing each day helps you savor the present moment. Life is a series of moments, and by being present and positive, you can fully appreciate and enjoy the beauty of the here and now.

- *Inspiration.* Your positivity and strength can serve as an inspiration to those around you. When you lead by example and show resilience, others may find the motivation to do the same in their lives.

- *Adaptability.* Life is unpredictable, and change is constant. Embracing positivity and strength enables you to adapt to new circumstances and challenges with a flexible and open mindset.

- *Sense of fulfillment.* Regaining control and embracing each day with positivity contributes to a deeper sense of fulfillment and purpose in life. They allow us to live with intention and appreciate the journey we are on.

Embracing positivity and strength does not mean ignoring or denying difficult emotions or challenges. Rather, it involves acknowledging these aspects of life while maintaining a constructive and optimistic perspective. Cultivating a positive mindset and inner strength is a continuous practice that requires self-awareness, self-compassion, and a willingness to learn and grow.

Ultimately, by regaining control over our lives and embracing positivity and strength, we can create a more joyful, fulfilling, and enriching life experience for ourselves and for those around us.

Taking responsibility for our mental health instead of blaming others or society for the level of unhappiness and frustration that we may experience is of paramount importance. We can choose to create a colorful and lovely garden of positive thoughts and beautiful imagery in our mind and attend it daily.

We need to be able to carefully select our thoughts, just like we pick flowers from a garden and view the external world through a perspective of self-awareness and appreciation. Cultivating positive thoughts and being able to regain control and master our reality could help us reject a life of feeling disempowered and devalued.

THE WORK-HOME BALANCE

Finding the right balance between work and personal time is crucial for maintaining good mental health and overall well-being.

This balance is essential for many reasons:

- *Preventing Burnout.* When work takes up too much time and energy, it can lead to burnout. Burnout is a state of emotional, physical, and mental exhaustion that results from chronic work-related stress. Having adequate personal time allows you to recharge.

- *Reducing stress.* A healthy work-life balance helps reduce overall stress levels. It allows you to engage in activities and hobbies that bring joy and relaxation, which are essential for managing and coping with stress.

- *Enhancing productivity.* Taking time on personal activities and relaxation can enhance your productivity at work. When you are well-rested and fulfilled outside of work, you are more focused and motivated when you are on the job.

- *Improving relationships.* Spending quality time with family and friends strengthens social connections and improves relationships. These meaningful connections provide emotional support and contribute to your overall happiness.

- *Promoting self-care.* Personal time allows you to prioritize self-care. Whether it's exercising, meditating, reading, or pursuing a hobby, these activities nourish our physical and mental well-being. Taking care of the way you look, improving the condition of your skin, and slowing down the aging process heal your mind and body while boosting the level of confidence and self-esteem.

- *Work satisfaction.* Creating a balance between work and personal life is a significant factor in job satisfaction. When you have time for personal interests and activities, you are more content and fulfilled in your professional role.

- *Boundary setting.* Establishing clear boundaries between work and personal life is essential for maintaining a healthy equilibrium. It prevents work from encroaching on your personal time and vice versa.

- *Overall happiness.* Striking a balance between work and personal life contributes to a higher overall level of happiness and life satisfaction. It allows you to lead a more fulfilling life beyond just your professional endeavors.

- *Long-term health.* Chronic imbalance between work and personal life can negatively impact your physical health over time. Stress-related health issues can arise if you neglect your personal well-being.

- *Setting a positive example.* Prioritizing work-life balance sets a positive example for others, whether they are colleagues, family members, or friends. It reinforces the importance of self-care and healthy boundaries in everyone's lives.

Work-life balance will look different for everyone, depending on personal circumstances and responsibilities. Striving for balance does not mean having equal hours devoted to work and personal life, but rather finding a harmony that allows us to meet our professional commitments while nurturing our personal needs and relationships. Communicating openly with employers, setting realistic expectations, and actively scheduling personal time are some strategies to achieve a healthier work-life balance. Taking steps toward this balance is an investment in our mental health, happiness, and long-term well-being.

MOVEMENT

A regular exercise routine will slow down the aging process, promote happiness, and help maintain a healthy body. In my clinical experience, patients confuse the concept of *activity* with *exercise*. Staying active is important at any age. For the activity to qualify as *exercise*, it will need to meet more stringent parameters.

While both staying active and engaging in exercise are valuable for overall health, they do have different implications and requirements.

Let's delve into the differences between the two:

Activity. Activity refers to any physical movement or task that expends energy. It encompasses a range of daily activities, such as walking, gardening, housekeeping, taking the stairs, playing with children or pets, and performing routine tasks at work. Staying active involves incorporating these activities into your daily life. Being physically active throughout the day contributes to improved circulation, increased energy expenditure, and enhanced overall well-being.

Exercise. Exercise, on the other hand, is a subset of physical activity that involves planned, structured, and repetitive movements with the specific purpose of improving physical fitness, strength, flexibility, or endurance. Unlike daily activities, exercise typically has predefined parameters, such as duration, intensity, and frequency. It often involves activities like jogging, weightlifting, cycling, yoga classes, or swimming. Exercise is deliberately performed to achieve certain fitness goals and requires a higher level of effort and commitment than everyday activities.

The main differences between activity and exercise lie in their structure, intention, and the degree of physical effort involved:

- *Structured versus unstructured.* Exercise involves planned and structured routines with specific exercises and repetitions, while activity is more spontaneous and can occur during daily tasks or leisure pursuits.

- *Specific goals.* Exercise is performed with the explicit purpose of improving fitness, strength, endurance, and flexibility or achieving specific health outcomes. Activity, while beneficial, might not have specific fitness goals.

- *Parameters.* Exercise adheres to defined parameters, such as metrics for changes in heart rate, calories burned, and shifts in strength, endurance, or weight. Everyday activity lacks these predetermined guidelines.

- *Intensity.* Exercise often involves higher levels of intensity and may push the body beyond the typical levels of activity experienced in daily life. Accelerated pulse, breathing, and sweating often occur during exercise.

- *Importance of both.* Staying active throughout the day, even in non-exercise activities, is vital for maintaining overall health, promoting circulation, and preventing sedentary behavior. Regular exercise, on the other hand, provides targeted benefits to different aspects of physical fitness and allows individuals to work on specific fitness goals.

In clinical practice, it's important to educate patients about the benefits of both staying active and engaging in structured exercise. I encourage patients to find opportunities for activity within their daily routines while emphasizing the value of incorporating planned exercise sessions to achieve optimal physical and mental well-being.

One of the parameters that defines an effective exercise regimen is to be able to reach and sustain your *target heart rate* for at least twenty minutes. The target heart rate is the range of heart beats per minute (bpm) at which your heart should ideally beat during aerobic exercise to maximize the benefits of the workout. The target heart rate is generally calculated based on a percentage of your maximum heart rate (MHR).

Achieving and sustaining your target heart rate helps you gauge the appropriate level of effort during aerobic or cardiovascular exercises to achieve your goals. The concept of target heart rate is often associated with moderate to vigorous aerobic activities.

To calculate your target heart rate, follow these steps:

1. **Determine Your Maximum Heart Rate (MHR)**: Subtract your age from 220. For example, if you are thirty years old, your estimated MHR would be

   220 - 30 = 190 bpm

2. **Choose the Intensity Level**: Depending on your fitness goals, select a target heart rate zone. For moderate-intensity exercise, aim for fifty to seventy percent of your MHR, while for vigorous-intensity exercise, aim for seventy to eighty-five percent of your MHR.

3. **Calculate Your Target Heart Rate Range**: Multiply your MHR by the desired percentage range.

   For example, if you want to exercise at a moderate intensity— sixty to seventy percent of MHR—and your MHR is 190 bpm, the target heart rate range would be 114–133 bpm.

   For a thirty-year-old individual aiming for moderate-intensity exercise—sixty to seventy percent of MHR:

MHR = 220 - 30 = 190 bpm

Target Heart Rate Range = 60%–70% of 190 bpm

Target Heart Rate Range = 114–133 bpm

Monitoring your heart rate during exercise can help ensure that you're working out at an appropriate level of intensity for the goal that you want to achieve.

Exercising within the target heart rate zone can:

- Improve cardiovascular fitness and endurance.

- Burn calories and aid in weight management.

- Enhance the efficiency of your workout by ensuring you're challenging your cardiovascular system appropriately.

- Reduce the risk of overexertion or injury during exercise.

Your target heart rate is a general guideline, and individual differences such as fitness level, health conditions, and medications may influence how your body responds to exercise. Always listen to your body and consult with a healthcare professional or fitness expert before starting or modifying an exercise program, especially if you have any health concerns or medical conditions.

SLEEP

According to the American Sleep Apnea Association, "About 50 to 70 million Americans have sleep disorders, and 1 in 3 adults (about 84 million people) do not regularly get the recommended amount of uninterrupted sleep that they need to protect their health."[28] (https://www.sleephealth.org)

A significant portion of the American population is sleep deprived. Sleep deprivation is a widespread issue that can have serious implications for physical health, cognitive function, mood, and overall well-being.

The *glymphatic system* is a recently discovered waste clearance pathway in the brain that plays a crucial role in removing metabolic waste products and toxins from the central nervous system. It was first identified and named in 2012 by researchers at the University of Rochester Medical Center.

The name *glymphatic* is a combination of *glial* and *lymphatic*. Glial cells are non-neuronal cells in the brain that provide support and protection to neurons, and the lymphatic system is a network of vessels and nodes that helps remove waste and immune cells from the body. The glymphatic system is primarily composed of glial cells, particularly a type called *astrocytes*, and is responsible for the clearance of waste products, including proteins like *beta-amyloid* and *tau*, which are associated with neurodegenerative diseases such as Alzheimer's disease.

The glymphatic system operates through the flow of cerebrospinal fluid (CSF) that moves through the brain tissue, facilitated by the expansion and contraction of brain cells during sleep. The discovery of the glymphatic system has highlighted the importance of sleep in promoting brain health and waste clearance, as the system appears to be most active during sleep.

Research into the glymphatic system is ongoing, and its full implications for brain health and disease are not yet fully understood. However, it has opened new avenues of study for understanding neurodegenerative disorders and has led to increased interest in investigating the impact of sleep on brain function and health.

Lack of sleep can have negative effects and can lead to cognitive impairment, mood disturbances, and even long-term health issues. So, while sleep does contribute to the removal of waste products from the brain, it's just one piece of the puzzle when it comes to the complex functions that sleep serves for overall brain health and bodily well-being.

Additional benefits of adequate, quality sleep include:

- *Memory consolidation and information processing.* During stages of sleep, the brain processes and organizes the information it has received from the environment and during the learning process. The deeper stages of non-REM (rapid eye movement) sleep are crucial for consolidating and strengthening memories. When you learn something new, your brain forms connections between different neurons. During sleep, these connections are reinforced and integrated into existing neural networks, which helps solidify the memory and make it more stable and accessible.

- *Enhanced learning process.* Sleep enhances your ability to extract important information from the day's experience and to make sense of complex information.

- *Processing and regulating emotional memories.* It can help reduce the emotional intensity of memories, making it easier to cope with overtime.

- *Creative thinking and problem-solving.* It's thought that during REM sleep, the brain combines information from various sources and explores novel connections, contributing to creative insights.

- *Spatial memory and navigation.* It helps consolidate memories related to the physical environment and spatial relationships.

- *Motor skill learning and coordination.* Sleep refines and consolidates the neural pathways involved in physical activities and movements.

Overall, sleep is a critical component of the learning and memory process, and getting adequate, quality sleep is essential for optimizing cognitive function, memory retention, and overall brain health.

Quality Sleep Maintains Health and Prevents Disease

During sleep, our body produces and releases *cytokines*, essential mediators that help fight infection, inflammation, and stress. A lack of sleep can weaken the immune system, making us more susceptible to infections and illnesses. Sleep has a significant impact on immune system function. T cells, a type of immune cell, are critical for immune response and inflammation control. Research suggests that sleep helps regulate the production and activity of T cells, contributing to proper immune function and reduced inflammation.

Lack of sleep can disrupt insulin sensitivity, increasing the risk of type 2 diabetes.

Sleep is important for maintaining the health of blood vessels. Poor sleep can lead to *endothelial dysfunction*, which is associated with increased inflammation and a higher risk of cardiovascular problems. Emerging research indicates that sleep can also influence the gut microbiome, the community of microorganisms living in the digestive tract. A balanced gut microbiome is crucial for immune function and inflammation regulation.

Sleep's Other Important Functions

Enhanced physical performance. Athletes and active individuals benefit from adequate sleep as it improves physical performance, coordination, and reaction time.

Cardiovascular health. Chronic sleep deprivation has been linked to an increased risk of heart disease, high blood pressure, and stroke. During deep sleep, blood pressure drops and the heart rate slows, allowing the cardiovascular system to rest and recover.

Weight management. Poor sleep can disrupt the balance of hunger-related hormones, such as ghrelin and leptin, leading to increased appetite and a higher likelihood of overeating. Chronic sleep deprivation has been associated with weight gain and obesity.

However, lack of sleep or poor-quality sleep can lead to the following effects on cortisol levels:

Elevated evening cortisol. Sleep deprivation or irregular sleep patterns can lead to elevated cortisol levels during the evening and night. This disruption can contribute to difficulty falling asleep, further exacerbating the sleep deficit.

Impaired suppression. Cortisol levels may not decrease as they should in the evening and during the night when sleep is compromised. This lack of suppression can lead to ongoing stress responses and potentially contribute to chronic stress.

Altered circadian rhythm. Sleep deprivation can disrupt the normal timing of cortisol secretion, leading to irregular patterns of cortisol release throughout the day.

Increased stress. Sleep deprivation itself is a stressor, and elevated cortisol levels are part of the body's response to stress. Chronically high cortisol levels due to inadequate sleep can contribute to a range of negative health outcomes, including increased risk of obesity, cardiovascular disease, and immune system dysfunction.

Metabolic effects. Elevated cortisol levels associated with sleep deprivation can also impact metabolism and insulin sensitivity, potentially leading to weight gain and an increased risk of type 2 diabetes.

Individual responses to sleep deprivation and cortisol regulation can vary. Chronic sleep deprivation and disruptions to cortisol rhythms can have cumulative negative effects on health over time.

Supporting Optimal Sleep Function

By prioritizing good sleep hygiene and getting enough rest, you can significantly enhance your overall health and reduce the risk of various diseases.

To ensure that sleep contributes positively to your health:

- Aim for seven to nine hours of sleep per night, as individual sleep needs may vary.

- Maintain a consistent sleep schedule by going to bed and waking up at the same time each day.

- Create a conducive sleep environment that is cool, dark, and quiet.

- Limit exposure to screens, blue light, and stimulating activities before bedtime.

- Avoid excessive caffeine and alcohol consumption, especially close to bedtime.

Sleep Cycles

Let's look at the physiology of sleep to better understand how it works and how to improve this fundamental body function.

Each sleep cycle typically lasts around 90 to 120 minutes and repeats multiple times throughout the night. The two main types of sleep are

Non-Rapid Eye Movement (NREM) sleep and Rapid Eye Movement (REM) sleep.

Let's explore each phase:

1. *NREM Stage 1 (N1).* This is the transition from wakefulness to sleep. It is a light sleep stage during which you may feel drowsy and relaxed. It is relatively easy to wake someone up during this stage, and muscle activity decreases.

2. *NREM Stage 2 (N2).* In this stage, the body further relaxes, and brain activity slows down. N2 sleep is characterized by the presence of *sleep spindles* and *K-complexes*—specific patterns of brain waves—on the electroencephalogram (EEG). These waves are thought to play a role in memory consolidation and protecting sleep stability.

3. *NREM Stage 3 (N3).* Also known as *slow-wave sleep* (SWS) or *deep sleep*, N3 is the most restorative stage of sleep. During this phase, the brain produces slow delta waves on the EEG. It is challenging to wake someone from deep sleep. If woken, they may feel groggy and disoriented. Deep sleep is crucial for physical recovery, growth, and boosting the immune system.

4. *REM Sleep.* After going through the NREM stages, the sleep cycle enters REM sleep, characterized by rapid eye movements, increased brain activity, and vivid dreams. During REM sleep, the body's muscles are mostly paralyzed to prevent acting out dreams. REM sleep is vital for memory consolidation, emotional regulation, and learning.

After REM sleep, the sleep cycle typically repeats itself, with each cycle comprising NREM and REM sleep in varying proportions. As the night progresses, the proportion of REM slcep increases, and deep sleep (N3) may decrease.

These sleep cycles are essential for achieving a well-rested and refreshed state. The different stages play unique roles in cognitive, emotional, and physical health. Disruptions to these sleep cycles, such as sleep disorders or inadequate sleep, can lead to various health problems and daytime impairment. It's crucial to prioritize sleep hygiene and establish a consistent sleep schedule to support healthy sleep cycles.

Sleep Monitoring

One way to make sure that the sleep has been restorative enough for the body is to monitor it. Monitoring your sleep can be a helpful way to identify any potential sleep issues or patterns that might be affecting your overall health and well-being. Sleep monitoring can provide valuable insights into the quality and duration of your sleep, helping you make necessary adjustments to improve your sleep hygiene and sleep habits.

Keeping a sleep diary involves manually recording details about your sleep patterns, such as the time you go to bed, the time you wake up, how long it takes you to fall asleep, and any potential disruptions during the night. You can also note factors like caffeine or alcohol consumption, exercise, blue light exposure, and stress levels to see how they may influence your sleep.

Here are some of the aids for monitoring sleep:

Wearable Sleep Trackers. Many fitness trackers and smartwatches come with built-in sleep tracking capabilities. These devices use sensors to monitor your movements, heart rate, and sometimes even respiratory rate during sleep. They provide data on sleep duration, sleep stages (NREM and REM), and the number of wakeful moments during the night.

I've been using "Whoop app" to track my sleep, monitor key health metrics, and analyze my daily activities, which has provided me with valuable insights to optimize my overall well-being.

- *Smartphone Apps*. Numerous smartphone apps are available that use your phone's sensors—e.g., accelerometer—to monitor your sleep patterns. Some of these apps analyze your movements during sleep to estimate sleep stages and provide sleep efficiency metrics.

- *Sleep Study (Polysomnography)*. If you suspect you have a significant sleep disorder, such as sleep apnea or narcolepsy, a sleep study conducted in a sleep clinic can provide detailed and accurate information about your sleep. This comprehensive test includes monitoring brain activity, eye movements, muscle activity, heart rate, and respiratory patterns.

By monitoring your sleep, you can identify trends and patterns that may be affecting the quality of your sleep, such as inconsistent bedtimes, excessive screen time before bed, or consuming stimulants too close to bedtime. Additionally, sleep monitoring can help you track improvements if you implement changes to your sleep routine or seek professional advice for sleep-related issues.

However, sleep monitoring is a complementary tool, and individual variations in sleep requirements can exist. If you consistently experience sleep difficulties, daytime fatigue, or other concerning symptoms, it's essential to consult a healthcare professional or a sleep specialist to identify and address any underlying sleep disorders or health issues.

They can provide personal recommendations and guidance based on a comprehensive assessment of your sleep health.

Another important consideration to understand the physiology of the sleep is the impact of the individual hormonal status.

Lack of hormonal balance found in women during perimenopause and after menopause can cause a profound disturbance of the sleep pattern.

The same can happen to men where a decrease in the level of essential gonadal hormones such as Testosterone, Pregnenolone and Progesterone can impact negatively in the quality of the sleep causing frequent awakenings or insomnia.

CHAPTER ELEVEN

ADAPTOGENS AND ALTERNATIVE THERAPIES

ADAPTOGENS

Adaptogens are natural substances believed to help the body adapt and respond better to stressors, including mental, physical, and emotional stress.

Herbal supplements classified as adaptogens may help promote a more restful sleep and support the body's response to stress. While they are not a substitute for healthy sleep habits, they may complement a well-rounded approach to improving sleep quality.

As with any herbal supplement, it's essential to consult with a healthcare professional before using these aids, especially if you are pregnant, nursing, or taking medications or have any underlying health conditions. Individual responses to herbal supplements may vary, and they may not be a substitute for medical treatment for specific health conditions. Always seek advice from a qualified healthcare professional for personal recommendations and guidance.

For example, chamomile may not be a good choice for those who suffer ragweed allergies, as it is a cousin to ragweed. Certain plants are powerful medicines that, taken over time, could pose adverse effects to kidneys, liver, or thyroid. Some of these substances are contraindicated in the presence of certain pharmaceuticals. So, it is vital that your choices for better health are thoroughly researched and guided by informed professionals.

Here are some popular adaptogens that are commonly used to support sleep:

Ashwagandha: Ashwagandha (*Withania sumnifera*), also known as winter cherry or Indian ginseng, is an herb used in traditional Ayurvedic medicine to help reduce stress, anxiety, and improve overall sleep quality. It is believed to have a calming effect on the nervous system.

Cannabis: Cannabis (genus in the family *Cannabaceae*) contains the component cannabidiol or CBD. Extracted into an oil, it has gained attention for its potential health benefits. Research is ongoing and more studies are needed to fully understand the mechanisms involved. CBD is believed to have anxiolytic (anxiety-reducing), anti-inflammatory, and analgesic (pain-relieving) properties. Reducing anxiety and chronic pain makes it easier for the body to rest.

CBD may influence the body's sleep-wake cycle by interacting with receptors in the endocannabinoid system, which plays a role in regulating various physiological processes. This interaction could help regulate the timing of sleep and wakefulness and may increase the duration of REM sleep.

CBD may help reduce disruptions during the night. CBD could promote relaxation and potentially address underlying issues that cause night-time awakenings, such as hypervigilance.

It's important to note that while CBD shows promise for sleep improvement, individual responses can vary and more research is needed to fully understand its effects on sleep. If you're considering using CBD oil to help with sleep, here are a few points to keep in mind:

- The appropriate dosage of CBD can vary widely among individuals. It's recommended to start with a low dose and gradually increase it if needed while monitoring its effects.

- Choose high-quality CBD oil from reputable manufacturers to ensure that you're getting a reliable product. Look for products that have been third-party tested for potency and purity.

- Before using CBD oil for sleep, especially if you have any underlying health conditions or are taking other medications, it's advisable to consult with a healthcare professional. They can provide personalized guidance based on your individual needs and circumstances.

- Consistency is key when using CBD oil for sleep improvement. Effects may not be immediate, and it may take some time for your body to respond.

In summary, CBD oil may offer potential benefits for sleep improvement by addressing anxiety, pain, and other factors that can interfere with restful sleep. However, it's important to approach its use with caution, consult a healthcare professional, and make informed decisions based on your individual needs and circumstances.

Chamomile: Chamomile (*Matricaria chamomilla*, *Chamaemelum nobile*, among several others) is a popular herbal remedy known for its calming properties. The dried flowers can be infused as a tea that is often used to help reduce stress and improve sleep quality.

Holy Basil: Holy basil (*Ocimum sanctum* or *Ocimum tenuiflorum*), also known as Tulsi, is an herb commonly used in traditional

Ayurvedic medicine. Holy basil can be consumed in various forms, including fresh herbs, dried leaves like teas or capsules, tinctures, and infused and essential oils. Holy basil tea is a popular and easy way to incorporate this herb into your daily routine. It is considered a sacred plant in India and has been revered for its medicinal properties for centuries. Holy basil contains compounds like flavonoids, polyphenols, and oils that have antioxidant and anti-inflammatory properties, which may contribute to its overall health benefits. Holy Basil is believed to support a healthy immune system and increase resistance to infections. It is also used to support digestive health and respiratory health, and address common respiratory conditions like coughs, colds, and bronchitis. While holy basil is generally considered safe for most people when consumed in typical culinary amounts, higher doses in supplement form may interact with certain medications or have potential side effects.

Lavender: The flowers and leaves of lavender (several species of the genus *Lavandula*), whether used as essential oil, tea, or ingested, are known for their relaxing and soothing effects. It is often used to promote a sense of calmness and improve sleep, as in sachets, potpourri, or aromatherapy as well as a culinary element.

Lemon Balm: Lemon balm (*Melissa officinalis*) is an herb with mild sedative properties that may help reduce anxiety and improve sleep.

Passionflower: Passionflower is another herb that may help improve sleep by reducing anxiety and inducing relaxation. It may also increase GABA levels, which contributes to its calming effects.

Rhodiola: Rhodiola (*Rhodiola rosea*) is not typically known for its sedative effects; however, Rhodiola rosea is considered an adaptogen that may help reduce stress and improve mental well-being, indirectly contributing to better sleep.

Melatonin: Melatonin is a hormone naturally produced by the pineal gland in the brain. It plays a crucial role in regulating the sleep-wake cycle, helping to signal to the body when it's time to sleep and when to wake up. Melatonin levels typically rise in the evening as it gets dark, promoting sleepiness, and decrease in the morning when it's time to wake up. As a supplement, melatonin is available in various forms, such as tablets, capsules, and gummies, and it is commonly used to address sleep-related issues, including insomnia and jet lag.

Melatonin can help shorten the time it takes to fall asleep, especially for people who have difficulty initiating sleep.

For individuals who work night shifts or irregular schedules, melatonin can aid in promoting sleep during nontraditional sleep times.

Melatonin is generally considered safe for short-term use when taken at appropriate dosages, but it's essential to use it responsibly and avoid long-term use without medical supervision. It's crucial to consult with a healthcare professional before starting melatonin supplements, especially for children, pregnant or nursing individuals, and those with certain medical conditions or taking medications.

While melatonin can be helpful for some individuals, it's important to remember that it is not a cure-all for sleep issues. Improving sleep hygiene, maintaining a consistent sleep schedule, managing stress, and creating a sleep-conducive environment are also essential factors in achieving restful and refreshing sleep.

Valerian: Valerian root has been used for centuries as a natural sleep aid. It is thought to enhance GABA (gamma-aminobutyric acid) levels in the brain, promoting relaxation and sleepiness. Valerian is available in various forms, such as capsules, teas, or extracts.

It's important to note that while these herbal supplements are generally considered safe, individual responses may vary. It's always a good idea to consult with a healthcare professional before starting any new supplements, especially if you are pregnant, nursing, taking medications, or have underlying health conditions.

Additionally, while adaptogens may help support stress reduction and potentially improve sleep quality, they are most effective when used in conjunction with a consistent sleep routine, proper sleep hygiene practices, and overall healthy lifestyle choices. If you are experiencing chronic sleep difficulties, it's essential to discuss your concerns with a healthcare provider or a sleep specialist to address any underlying issues properly.

LIGHT THERAPY

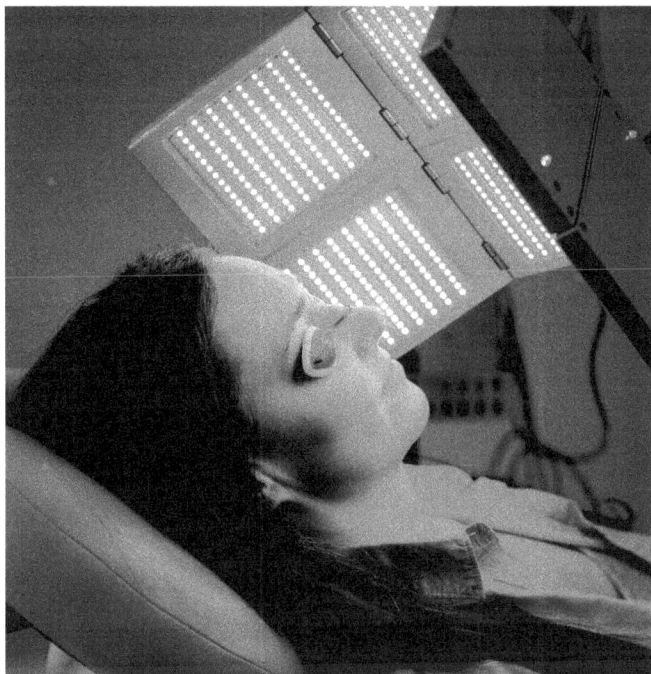

Light therapy, also known as *phototherapy* or *bright light therapy*, uses combined red, infrared, and UV light to treat various conditions and improve overall well-being. It is commonly used to treat seasonal affective disorder (SAD) and sleep disorders, but it has several other benefits as well.

I have been using "Lightwave therapy" for myself and for my patients for several years and I am a firm believer in the positive effects on body and mind.

Here are some of the benefits of light therapy:

Alleviates depression. SAD is a type of depression that occurs during specific seasons, most commonly in the fall and winter when there is less natural sunlight. Regular exposure to bright light can help alleviate the symptoms of SAD, such as low mood, fatigue, and changes in sleep patterns.

Regulates circadian rhythms. Exposure to bright light, particularly in the morning, helps regulate the body's internal clock, known as the *circadian rhythm.* This can improve sleep patterns, making it beneficial for individuals with insomnia or other sleep disorders.

Enhances mood. Light therapy has been shown to have positive effects on mood and emotional well-being beyond treating SAD. It can help improve feelings of depression and anxiety in some individuals.

Assists in adjusting to jet lag and shift work. Light therapy can aid in adjusting to new time zones and managing the disruptions caused by jet lag. Additionally, it can be helpful for individuals who work night shifts by helping them adapt their internal clock to their work schedule.

Heightens energy and alertness. Regular exposure to bright light can increase energy levels and alertness, making it helpful for individuals who experience lethargy or drowsiness during the day.

Improves skin condition. Light therapy can be used to treat certain skin conditions like psoriasis, eczema, and acne. Different wavelengths of light are used for these treatments to target specific skin issues.

Stabilizes seasonal variations in bipolar disorder. Some research suggests that light therapy may help stabilize mood and reduce depressive symptoms in certain individuals with bipolar disorder, particularly during specific seasons.

Can address behavioral changes. There is some evidence to suggest that light therapy might have potential benefits in managing behavioral disturbances in individuals with dementia and Alzheimer's disease.

Offers noninvasive, safe options for treatment. Light therapy is generally considered safe when used correctly and under the guidance of a healthcare professional. It is noninvasive and does not involve the use of medications, reducing the risk of side effects.

Light therapy can be beneficial for many people; however, it may not be suitable for everyone, and individual responses can vary. Consulting with a healthcare professional is essential to determine the most appropriate treatment plan and to ensure that it is safe and effective for a specific condition.

EASTERN-INFLUENCED TREATMENT MODALITIES

Acupuncture

Acupuncture is a form of alternative medicine that has been practiced for thousands of years. Its origins can be traced back to ancient China, and it is believed to have been developed around five thousand years ago, though some historical evidence suggests it may be even older. The practice of acupuncture involves inserting thin needles into specific points on the body to stimulate various physiological responses.

The primary goal of acupuncture is to restore the balance of energy, known as *qi* or *chi* (pronounced *chee*), within the body. In traditional Chinese medicine (TCM), it is believed that imbalances in the flow of qi can lead to disease and health problems. By targeting specific points along the energy pathways in the body, practitioners aim to promote the smooth flow of qi and restore harmony.

Acupuncture is often used as a holistic approach to treat various health conditions and promote overall well-being. While it has been historically used for disease prevention, it is also utilized to address existing ailments and alleviate symptoms such as pain, stress, anxiety, and digestive issues. Its philosophy stresses the importance of establishing balanced communication among the vital organs in the body along energy pathways known as *meridians*.

TCM philosophy takes a holistic approach to health, viewing the body as an integrated whole rather than a collection of isolated parts. It emphasizes the interconnection between different organs, systems, and the external environment and teaches the importance of finding a balance for humans within nature. Each organ can interact and communicate with other organs like a symphony. One system affects all others. When the energetic field of one organ is imbalanced because of a lack of the normal flow of the chi, it creates a fertile ground for a disease to establish.

Some diseases are caused by an excess of stagnant energy that can interfere with the normal function of the organ affected. The same is true in cases of intrinsic deficiency of the qi. Along the meridians are *acupoints*, which are points where the flow of qi can be accessed and manipulated. When the flow of qi is balanced and unobstructed, the body is in a state of health. If there is a blockage or imbalance in the flow of qi, it can lead to illness and disease.

Acupuncture philosophy also incorporates the concept of *Yin and Yang*, which represent opposing and complementary forces in nature, such as rest and activity, masculine and feminine, dark and light. The balance between Yin and Yang is essential for maintaining health. When Yin and Yang are in harmony, the body is in a state of balance. Imbalances between Yin and Yang can lead to various health issues.

Acupuncture treatments are highly individualized, and practitioners consider a person's overall health, lifestyle, and specific symptoms before formulating a treatment plan. The goal is to restore the balance of qi and promote the body's natural healing abilities.

Acupuncture is not only used for treating existing health problems but is also considered a preventive measure to maintain overall health and prevent future illnesses by keeping the qi flow balanced. This represents one of the most powerful and modern meanings that has immense value in today's world and environment.

Over time, acupuncture has gained popularity and acceptance worldwide, and its practice has evolved to incorporate modern medical knowledge and research. Many people find relief and benefits from acupuncture treatments.

Some health insurance plans in the U.S. even include coverage for acupuncture to mitigate pain after surgery or nausea due to cancer treatments.

Feng Shui

Feng shui (pronounced *fung shway*) is an ancient Chinese practice that seeks to harmonize and balance qi in the environment to promote health, wealth, and well-being. It is considered an art and a science that dates back thousands of years and is deeply rooted in Chinese culture and philosophy.

The term *feng shui* translates to wind (feng) and water (shui), reflecting the idea of harnessing the natural elements to create a positive energy flow. The practice is based on the belief that the arrangement and orientation of objects and spaces can influence the flow of energy, and thus affect the health, wealth, and happiness of those who live or work in the environment.

Key principles of feng shui include:

- *Bagua.* The bagua is a fundamental concept in feng shui that divides a space into nine areas or zones, each representing a different aspect of life, such as wealth, career, family, health, and relationships. By understanding the bagua, practitioners can assess the energy in specific areas and adjust to enhance the corresponding aspects of life.

- *Five elements.* Feng shui incorporates the five elements— Wood, Fire, Earth, Metal, and Water—which are believed to interact with each other and influence the energy of space. These elements are often represented through colors, shapes, and materials to create a harmonious balance.

- *Yin and Yang.* Feng shui considers the concept of Yin and Yang, representing complementary forces and opposite energies. Balancing these forces within a space is thought to be vital for creating harmony and promoting positive energy flow.

- *Cardinal directions.* The compass plays a crucial role in traditional feng shui, as practitioners use it to determine the best orientation and arrangement of a space to harness positive energy and minimize negative influences.

Feng shui is applied to various aspects of life, including home and office design, interior decoration, landscaping, and city planning.

It is widely practiced in many parts of the world, with the aim of creating a balanced and harmonious environment that fosters well-being and prosperity. However, it is essential to note that while many people believe in the benefits of feng shui, its principles and effectiveness remain a matter of personal belief and cultural tradition.

CHAPTER TWELVE

THE AGING PROCESS

We are programmed to die. This is our biological destiny. The aging process starts at birth. Our biological lifespan is dictated by the length of our chromosomes. The shorter the chromosomes, the shorter our lifespan.

TELOMERES AND TELOMERASE

The length of our chromosomes is regulated by the presence of a sequence structure called telomeres, first mentioned in Chapter Five. To review, telomeres are repetitive sequences of DNA located at the ends of chromosomes. Their primary function is to protect the genetic information within the chromosome from degradation and from fusing with neighboring chromosomes. Think of telomeres as the protective tips on shoelaces that maintain the integrity of chromosome ends, ensuring they don't wear out over time.

As cells divide, their telomeres naturally shorten. This is due to the inherent limitations of DNA replication machinery and the end replication problem. In most somatic (body) cells, the enzyme telomerase is not very active or is completely absent.

Telomerase is a specialized reverse transcriptase enzyme that can add back telomere sequences to the ends of chromosomes, effectively counteracting the shortening process. The reason telomerase is not very active in most somatic cells is closely tied to the balance between cell division and the potential for cancer. Unregulated activation of telomerase can lead to cells dividing uncontrollably, which is a hallmark of cancer. In contrast, germ cells (sperm and egg cells) and some stem cells have higher levels of telomerase activity, allowing them to maintain their telomere length and divide more extensively.

The Hayflick limit is the phenomenon in which cells have a limited number of divisions before they enter a state of replicative senescence, essentially halting their ability to divide further. Telomere shortening plays a role in this process, but it's not the only factor.

The relationship between telomeres, telomerase, aging, and cancer is complex and still an active area of research. Some studies suggest that telomere length can be influenced by various lifestyle factors such as stress, diet, exercise, and overall health. Researchers are also investigating the potential therapeutic applications of targeting telomerase in cancer treatment and exploring ways to potentially extend a healthy lifespan by modulating telomere maintenance.

Astragalus and Telomerase

While there is ongoing research on the potential health benefits of astragalus and its compounds, including the possibility of telomere protection, the direct claim that astragalus blocks the effect of telomerase and prolongs human lifespan is not firmly established. Some studies suggest that certain compounds found in astragalus may have anti-aging or protective effects on cells, but more research is needed to fully understand their mechanisms and potential applications in humans.

Viruses, Cancer, and Immortalization

Human Papillomavirus (HPV) and certain cancerous cells do indeed exhibit the ability to produce oncoproteins that contribute to cellular immortalization. These oncoproteins interfere with normal cell cycle regulation and can promote uncontrolled cell division. HPV oncoproteins, for instance, are known to interfere with the function of tumor suppressor proteins like p53.

Telomerase and Immortalization

Telomerase is associated with cellular immortalization. In some cases, cancer cells can reactivate telomerase, allowing them to maintain or even lengthen their telomeres, which helps them evade the Hayflick limit and continue dividing indefinitely. This contributes to the unchecked growth and spread of cancer cells.

Furthermore, the relationship between telomerase, cellular immortalization, and cancer is complex and varies depending on the context. Some cancers rely on telomerase activation, while others use alternative mechanisms to maintain telomere length. Researchers are actively studying these processes to develop better strategies for cancer treatment and understanding cellular aging.

HORMONES

The aging process is associated with changes in hormone production and regulation within the body.

Hormones are chemical messengers that play a crucial role in regulating various processes and functions within the body. They are produced by specialized glands, such as the pituitary gland, thyroid gland, adrenal glands, and more. These hormones travel through the bloodstream to reach their target organs or tissues, where they exert their effects by binding to specific receptors. Hormones are responsible for maintaining *homeostasis*, which is the balance of internal conditions required for the body to function properly.

They regulate a wide range of physiological processes, including:

- *Metabolism.* Hormones like insulin, produced by the pancreas, regulate glucose metabolism and play a role in maintaining stable blood sugar levels.

- *Growth and development.* Hormones like growth hormone and thyroid hormones influence growth, development, and maturation of various tissues and organs.

- *Reproduction and Sexual Function.* Hormones such as estrogen and testosterone are vital for reproductive processes, sexual development, and maintenance of secondary sexual characteristics.

- *Stress Response.* Hormones like cortisol, released by the adrenal glands, help the body respond to stress and regulate various metabolic activities.

- *Immune System Regulation.* Some hormones have immunomodulatory effects, influencing the body's immune response to infections and other challenges.

- *Fluid and electrolyte balance.* Hormones like aldosterone regulate fluid and electrolyte balance in the body.

- *Mood and emotions.* Hormones such as serotonin and dopamine can influence mood, emotions, and overall mental well-being.

- *Bone Health.* Hormones like parathyroid hormone and calcitonin help regulate calcium levels and bone health.

- *Thermoregulation.* Hormones play a role in maintaining body temperature within a narrow range.

- *Sleep.* Hormones like melatonin help regulate the body's internal clock and sleep-wake cycles.

These are just a few examples of the many functions that hormones control. The precise balance and interactions between different hormones are essential for the proper functioning of the body's systems. Any disruption in hormone production, release, or receptor sensitivity can lead to various health issues and imbalances.

The aging process in both sexes will translate into the deficiency of the hormones that are produced by our gonads. Estrogen and progesterone levels in women and progesterone plus testosterone levels in men decline over time.

Menopause in women and andropause in men can be considered a hormonal imbalance caused by the considerable decline in the production and the release of the sexual hormones in the blood stream.

Menopause is a natural biological process that marks the end of a woman's reproductive years. It is characterized by a significant decline in the production of estrogen and progesterone, which are primarily produced by the ovaries.

During menopause, the ovaries gradually stop releasing eggs, and the menstrual cycle becomes irregular before eventually ceasing altogether. This hormonal transition can lead to a range of physical and emotional changes, and many of the symptoms experienced during menopause are a result of the hormonal fluctuations and imbalances that occur.

Some common symptoms of menopause include:

- *Hot flashes and night sweats.* Sudden and intense feelings of warmth, often accompanied by sweating, can disrupt sleep and daily activities.

- *Mood changes.* Fluctuations in hormone levels can contribute to mood swings, irritability, and feelings of sadness or anxiety.

- *Vaginal changes.* Lower estrogen levels can lead to vaginal dryness, vaginal atrophy, changes in the epithelial cells of the vaginal canal, discomfort during intercourse, and a change in the pH of the vaginal microbiome, which can mean an increased risk of urinary tract infections and yeast infections.

- *Sleep disturbances.* Hormonal changes can impact sleep patterns and contribute to insomnia or disrupted sleep. The ability to have a good quality sleep becomes impaired with more superficial sleep and frequent awakening episodes during the night with the result of poor energy level, decreased endurance, mood swings with irritability and decreased memory.

- *Changes in libido.* Reduced hormone levels can lead to changes in sexual desire and function.

- *Bone health.* Estrogen plays a role in maintaining bone density, so its decline during menopause can increase the risk of osteoporosis, potential for greater risk of bone breaks, and other conditions.

- *Cognitive changes.* Some women may experience changes in memory, concentration, or cognitive function during menopause.

- *Weight changes.* Hormonal fluctuations can contribute to changes in body composition and weight distribution. Slowly but steadily, our muscle mass starts decreasing around age thirty, and it accelerates the process at an exponential rate at the time of menopause/andropause because of such a lack of gonadal hormones. We are not able to grow muscles as before even with the same level of exercise; therefore, muscles are replaced with fat. The body shape changes with more fat deposition in the middle section; our metabolism slows down, causing more weight gain.

- *Cardiovascular changes.* Estrogen has protective effects on the cardiovascular system, and its decline can influence heart health. Bad cholesterol and triglyceride levels start climbing after menopause, causing the narrowing of the blood vessels that further decreases the blood flow to vital organs such as our brain and the heart.

- *Skin and hair changes.* Hormonal imbalances can impact skin elasticity, moisture levels, and hair texture.

Testosterone is the primary male sex hormone and plays a crucial role in the development and maintenance of male reproductive tissues, as well as the regulation of various physiological functions. As men age, their testosterone levels naturally decrease, and this decline can lead to a range of physical, emotional, and cognitive changes. Andropause is also sometimes referred to as *male menopause* or *late-onset hypogonadism.* It is a natural and gradual process that typically occurs around the age of forty or fifty. However, unlike menopause in women, which involves a significant and relatively rapid decline in hormone levels, the hormonal changes in andropause are more gradual and less pronounced.

Some potential symptoms of andropause include:

- *Decreased energy levels.* Men may experience fatigue, reduced stamina, and a decrease in overall energy levels.

- *Changes in mood.* Mood swings, irritability, and feelings of depression or anxiety may occur.

- *Reduced sexual function.* Lower testosterone levels can lead to decreased libido (sex drive), erectile dysfunction, and changes in sexual performance.

- *Changes in body composition.* Muscle mass may decrease, while body fat may increase. This can lead to changes in body composition and overall strength.

- *Sleep disturbances.* Insomnia or disrupted sleep patterns may become more common.

- *Cognitive changes*. Some men may experience changes in memory, concentration, and cognitive function.

- *Bone health*. Reduced testosterone levels can contribute to a gradual decrease in bone density and an increased risk of osteoporosis. Bones become more brittle because of the enhanced process of demineralization and bone reabsorption, which is no longer prevented by the presence of sexual hormones. Unable to grow new bones, we become more prone to fractures, which can cause significant morbidity and increased overall mortality.

- *Hair and skin changes*. Changes in hair growth patterns and skin texture may occur.

- *Cardiovascular Health*. Some research suggests a potential link between low testosterone levels and cardiovascular health. This is due to a higher risk of developing metabolic syndrome, with impaired lipid metabolism and an increase in fat deposition in the body.

Not all men will experience significant symptoms of andropause, and the severity of symptoms can vary widely among individuals. Moreover, the symptoms of andropause can overlap with other medical conditions or lifestyle factors. If a man is experiencing symptoms that may be related to andropause, it's advisable to consult with a healthcare professional. A doctor can evaluate symptoms, perform appropriate tests, and recommend potential interventions, which may include lifestyle changes, hormone replacement therapy, or other treatments based on individual needs.

While it is true that the decline in sex hormone production can impact the functioning of different systems and organs in the body, aging is a multifaceted process influenced by a combination of genetic, environmental, and lifestyle factors. Hormone deficiencies can contribute to certain age-related changes, but they are just one component of the larger picture.

I've been relying on a lab called "Genova" to assess both metabolic and hormonal profiles in patients with complex cases. This approach has helped me uncover key insights and recommend targeted adjustments to their therapy, diet, and exercise, ultimately enhancing their health and optimizing their performance.

THE IMPACT OF POOR SLEEP

Poor sleep can have a significant impact on the aging process, both in terms of accelerating certain aspects of aging and contributing to various age-related health issues. The quality of sleep can indeed be affected by various factors, including hormonal changes, as we age. Hormones like melatonin and cortisol play a crucial role in regulating our sleep-wake cycles, and disruptions in their production and balance can lead to problems with the ability to sleep.

As people age, there can be changes in their circadian rhythm, which is the internal clock that regulates the sleep-wake cycle. These changes can lead to more fragmented and lighter sleep, making it difficult to achieve the deeper, restorative stages of sleep. This can result in frequent awakenings during the night, more superficial sleep, and an overall decrease in sleep quality.

The consequences of poor sleep quality can be far-reaching and impact various aspects of daily life, causing decreased energy levels, reduced endurance, mood swings with irritability, and impaired memory. Inadequate sleep and sleep disturbances can also contribute to a higher risk of various health conditions, including cardiovascular diseases, metabolic disorders, and cognitive decline.

Here are some ways in which poor sleep can affect aging:

- *Cellular aging.* Sleep is crucial for cellular repair and maintenance. Poor sleep can disrupt these processes, leading to accelerated cellular aging. This can manifest as a decrease in the length of telomeres, which are protective caps at the end of chromosomes. Shorter telomeres are associated with increased cellular aging and a higher risk of age-related diseases.

- *Cognitive decline.* Chronic sleep deprivation and poor sleep quality are linked to cognitive decline and an increased risk of neurodegenerative diseases such as Alzheimer's and Parkinson's. During deep sleep stages, the brain clears out toxins and metabolic waste products that accumulate throughout the day. Inadequate sleep can hinder this waste clearance process and contribute to cognitive impairment.

- *Physical health issues.* Poor sleep is associated with a higher risk of various physical health problems that become more prevalent with age, such as cardiovascular disease, diabetes, obesity, and hypertension. Sleep helps regulate hormones and processes that are crucial for maintaining overall health. Disruption of these processes due to poor sleep can contribute to the development of these age-related conditions.

- *Immune function.* Sleep plays a vital role in supporting the immune system. Inadequate sleep can weaken the immune response, making older adults more susceptible to infections and potentially delaying recovery from illnesses.

- *Inflammation.* Poor sleep is associated with chronic low-grade inflammation, which is a hallmark of the aging process and is linked to various age-related diseases, including heart disease, diabetes, and certain cancers.

- *Skin aging.* Sleep is important for skin health and regeneration. Lack of sleep can lead to increased skin aging, including the appearance of fine lines, wrinkles, and uneven skin tone.

- *Mood and mental health.* Sleep disturbances are closely tied to mood disorders such as depression and anxiety, which can affect the quality of life and contribute to an accelerated aging process.

- *Hormonal imbalance.* Sleep is crucial for maintaining a healthy balance of hormones, including those that regulate stress (cortisol) and growth (growth hormone). Disruption in these hormonal patterns due to poor sleep can impact overall well-being and aging. Sex hormonal deficiency can have a significant negative impact in the quality of the sleep.

- *Metabolic effects.* Poor sleep can lead to disruptions in metabolism, including insulin resistance and impaired glucose tolerance. These metabolic changes are associated with an increased risk of age-related diseases like type 2 diabetes.

Making positive changes to sleep habits and addressing sleep-related issues can potentially slow down or mitigate some of these effects. Practicing good sleep hygiene, managing stress, maintaining a healthy lifestyle, and seeking medical advice for sleep disorders can all contribute to healthier aging.

Maintaining good *sleep hygiene* practices includes creating a comfortable, cooler sleep environment, establishing a regular sleep schedule, avoiding stimulants before bedtime, and managing stress. In some cases, medical interventions, including hormone replacement therapy (HRT) or other treatments, may be considered to address sleep-related issues associated with hormonal changes.

Empower Your Health

OXIDATIVE STRESS AND THE AGING PROCESS

Oxidative stress is a term used to describe an imbalance between the production of *reactive oxygen species* (ROS), also known as *free radicals*, and the body's ability to neutralize and detoxify them using antioxidants. Reactive oxygen species are highly reactive molecules containing oxygen that are generated as natural byproducts of various metabolic processes within cells, including energy production.

In moderate amounts, ROS plays an important role in cell signaling, immune response, and various physiological functions. However, excessive ROS production can lead to damage to cellular components such as DNA, proteins, and lipids. This damage, in turn, can contribute to various diseases, including neurodegenerative disorders, cardiovascular diseases, and cancer as well as the aging process.

As it pertains to aging, oxidative stress is believed to play a significant role in the gradual deterioration of cellular function and the overall aging of the body.

Here's how oxidative stress is thought to contribute to the aging process:

1. *Cellular damage.* Over time, the accumulation of oxidative damage to cellular components can impair the normal functioning of cells. For example, oxidative damage to DNA can lead to mutations, oxidative damage to proteins can disrupt their structure and function, and oxidative damage to lipids can result in inflammation and other negative effects.

2. *Mitochondrial dysfunction.* Mitochondria are the powerhouses of cells and are responsible for energy production. They are particularly susceptible to oxidative stress because of their role in producing energy and the presence of ROS as byproducts of this process. Accumulated oxidative damage to mitochondrial

DNA and proteins can lead to mitochondrial dysfunction, reducing energy production and accelerating the aging process.

3. *Inflammation.* Oxidative stress can trigger an inflammatory response in the body. Chronic inflammation, driven in part by oxidative stress, is associated with a variety of age-related diseases and can contribute to tissue damage and dysfunction.

4. *Cellular senescence.* Oxidative stress has been linked to the process of cellular senescence, in which cells lose their ability to divide and function properly. Senescent cells can accumulate in tissues and contribute to various age-related conditions.

5. *Telomere shortening.* Telomeres are protective caps on the ends of chromosomes that shorten with each cell division. Oxidative stress and inflammation are thought to accelerate telomere shortening, which is associated with cellular aging and overall aging of the organism.

To counteract the negative effects of oxidative stress, the body relies on antioxidants. Antioxidants are molecules that neutralize ROS and prevent them from causing damage. The body produces its own antioxidants, and they can also be obtained from dietary sources such as fruits, vegetables, and certain supplements.

While oxidative stress is considered a significant contributor to the aging process, aging is a complex and multifaceted phenomenon influenced by a variety of genetic, environmental, and lifestyle factors. Researchers continue to investigate the exact mechanisms through which oxidative stress impacts aging and to explore potential interventions to mitigate its effects.

AGING AND THE IMMUNE SYSTEM

A robust and well-functioning immune system contributes to an extended lifespan by decelerating the aging process. The connection between the vitality of our immune system and the pace of our biological aging becomes evident through the examination of certain illnesses.

The impact of certain diseases on our immune system's well-being becomes strikingly apparent in how they influence our biological aging. A noteworthy example is the accelerated aging observed in individuals who have AIDS.

In the natural course of the disease, some patients exhibit premature aging, appearing twenty to thirty years older than their chronological age by the time of their passing.

HIV selectively attacks immune cells, leading to immune system dysfunction and debilitation. When patients with HIV have not received proper medical intervention, the aging process seems to advance rapidly, manifesting in accelerated deterioration of the skin, hair, muscles, and skeletal structure.

We've come to realize that our immune system serves not only as a safeguard against external threats, but also as a key orchestrator in the intricate process of aging. Our dietary choices hold a profound significance beyond mere fulfillment of cravings or hunger pangs; they play a pivotal role in nurturing a robust immune system.

Indeed, our diet wields considerable influence over the health of our immune system, as well as the optimal functioning of our brain and body.

A poor diet high in excessive sugar, processed foods, and genetically modified products heightens inflammation within our bodies.

This hastens the aging trajectory and increases the susceptibility to a range of ailments including hypertension, diabetes, arthritis, and autoimmune conditions such as rheumatoid arthritis, lupus (LES), and Hashimoto's disease. The spectrum of potential maladies extends to Alzheimer's, cancer, and more.

Moreover, the inflammatory shifts within our bodily systems can even induce modifications in the expression of our genes within the DNA, escalating the likelihood of mutations and ultimately fostering a terrain conducive to cancer.

The paramount importance of adhering to a diet brimming with fresh, organically sourced vegetables and fruit, pasture-raised animals, and grass-fed beef is universally acknowledged. Concomitantly, curbing consumption of dairy products and processed foods resonates as a prudent approach.

We must consider the potential for cumulative toxic overload in the body over time, especially as the body's ability to efficiently clear toxins and chemicals may decrease with aging.

Toxins and chemicals can enter the body through various sources, such as the environment, food, water, air, and personal care products.

Over time, these substances can accumulate in tissues and organs, potentially leading to health issues. The body has natural detoxification processes, primarily carried out by the liver, kidneys, and skin, which help eliminate these substances. However, as the body ages, these processes may become less efficient, leading to a slower clearance of toxins.

This can contribute to a variety of health problems, including chronic diseases, cognitive decline, and compromised immune function. It's important for individuals, especially as they age, to take steps to minimize their exposure to toxins and support their body's natural detoxification processes.

This can include adopting a healthy diet, staying hydrated, engaging in regular exercise, managing stress, and avoiding or minimizing exposure to environmental toxins whenever possible.

While the concept of cumulative toxic overload is valid, the extent of its impact on individual health can vary greatly depending on factors such as genetics, lifestyle choices, and environmental exposures. As our understanding of toxicology and its effects on the aging body continues to evolve, researchers and healthcare professionals can provide more targeted guidance for mitigating potential risks associated with cumulative toxin exposure.

Toxins and cancer-promoting factors, such as the ones produced by smoking cigarettes and cigars, increase the risk of mouth cancer, cervical cancer, lung cancer, and bladder cancer.

Some heavy metals and dyes, preservatives, fertilizers, and GMO food can have carcinogenic effects on our body from directly damaging our DNA and/or triggering an inflammatory response that can weaken our immune system function.

Exposure to these chemicals needs to be avoided.

CHAPTER THIRTEEN

STRESS AND AGING

Aging can bring about positive changes, such as increased wisdom, resilience, and a more relaxed attitude toward life. However, some aspects of aging create stress or anxiety in many individuals.

Stress can accelerate the aging process through various biological mechanisms that impact the body's cells and systems. Here are some key ways stress contributes to aging:

Telomere Shortening

Telomeres are protective caps at the ends of chromosomes that prevent genetic material from deteriorating. Chronic stress can lead to faster shortening of telomeres, which is associated with accelerated cellular aging and increased risk of age-related diseases.

Oxidative Stress

Stress increases the production of free radicals, unstable molecules that can damage cells. This oxidative stress can harm DNA, proteins, and cell membranes, leading to premature cellular aging and dysfunction.

Inflammation

Chronic stress triggers a prolonged inflammatory response. While acute inflammation helps heal wounds, chronic inflammation can damage tissues and organs, contributing to the aging process and the development of age-related conditions such as cardiovascular disease and arthritis.

Hormonal Imbalance

Stress activates the hypothalamic-pituitary-adrenal (HPA) axis, leading to the release of stress hormones like cortisol. Prolonged high levels of cortisol can weaken the immune system, increase blood pressure, and promote the breakdown of muscle and bone, all associated with aging.

Impact on Skin

Stress can negatively affect the skin by reducing its ability to retain moisture, accelerating the breakdown of collagen and increasing the formation of wrinkles. Stress-related habits like poor sleep and unhealthy eating can also impact skin health.

Impact on Sleep

Stress often disrupts sleep patterns, leading to insufficient or poor-quality sleep. Chronic sleep deprivation is linked to a variety of health issues, including impaired cognitive function, decreased immune response, and increased risk of chronic diseases, and all contribute to aging.

Metabolic Changes

Chronic stress can lead to metabolic imbalances, including insulin resistance and increased abdominal fat. These metabolic changes are risk factors for diabetes, cardiovascular disease, and other age-related conditions.

Behavioral Changes

Stress can lead to unhealthy behaviors, such as smoking, excessive alcohol consumption, poor diet, and lack of exercise. These behaviors can further contribute to the aging process and the development of chronic diseases.

Several factors contribute to the potential for increased stress and anxiety with age:

- *Life changes.* As people age, they often go through significant life changes, such as retirement, health issues, loss of loved ones, or financial concerns. These changes can bring about stressors that may lead to increased anxiety.

- *Physical health.* Aging can bring about various physical health challenges, and dealing with chronic illnesses or pain can contribute to stress and anxiety.

- *Cognitive changes.* Cognitive changes and memory decline that can occur with aging may lead to concerns about cognitive function, which can be anxiety-inducing.

- *Social isolation.* As people get older, they may become more socially isolated due to factors such as retirement, loss of friends and family members, or limited mobility. Social isolation can contribute to feelings of loneliness and anxiety.

- *Adjusting to a new role.* Retirement and the transition from a career-oriented life to a more leisure-focused one can lead to a loss of identity and purpose.

- *Financial concerns.* Many individuals worry about financial stability during retirement, especially if they haven't adequately prepared.

- *Mental health awareness.* With increased awareness and reduced stigma around mental health, older individuals may be more likely to recognize and seek help for their stress and anxiety.

RELIEVING STRESS

Many older adults find effective ways to manage stress and anxiety, such as staying socially engaged, practicing relaxation techniques, engaging in physical activity, seeking professional support when needed, and maintaining a positive outlook.

Consistent practice of yoga and meditation can be beneficial for managing stress and promoting overall well-being, regardless of age. Both practices have been shown to have positive effects on mental and physical health.

Here's how they can help:

Yoga

- *Physical benefits.* Yoga involves various postures, stretches, and breathing exercises that can help improve flexibility, strength, and balance. Engaging in physical activity has been linked to the release of endorphins, which are natural mood lifters.

- *Relaxation.* Many yoga practices emphasize relaxation and stress reduction. Techniques like deep breathing and progressive muscle relaxation incorporated into yoga sessions can help calm the nervous system and reduce stress levels.

- *Mindfulness.* Yoga encourages mindfulness and being present in the moment, meaning being able to pay attention to whatever is happening in the body, moment by moment, while being able to remove distractions, worries, and other parasitic thoughts that will interfere with the process. This can help redirect your focus away from stressors and anxieties, promoting a sense of mental clarity and peace.

Meditation

- *Stress reduction.* Meditation techniques, such as mindfulness meditation and loving-kindness meditation, have been shown to reduce stress and anxiety by promoting relaxation and reducing the body's physiological responses to stress.

- *Emotional regulation.* Regular meditation practice can help you become more aware of your thoughts and emotions, allowing you to respond to them in a more balanced and constructive manner.

- *Cognitive benefits.* Meditation has been associated with improved cognitive function, including enhanced attention, focus, and memory. This can contribute to better stress management and overall mental well-being.

Combining Yoga and Meditation

The combination of yoga and meditation can be particularly powerful for stress management. Yoga provides a physical outlet for stress while also incorporating mindful awareness of the body and breath. Meditation deepens this mindfulness and can help you become more attuned to your mental and emotional states.

Of course, the efficacy of these practices varies for individuals, dependent on many factors. Consistency is key; regular practice over time is more likely to yield positive results. If you're new to yoga or meditation, consider starting with beginner-friendly classes or guided sessions to learn proper techniques.

Creating a happy, comfortable, and safe place inside us is important to keep our emotional balance. We need to learn how to shield our minds from the harmful effects of negative emotions and toxic information as well as the harsh environment. We need to practice the ability of creating stillness in our minds.

Focus on the Moment

Pay attention to your body and learn to read the subtle messages that lie within. The ability to quiet our mind and listen to our body is essential to maintaining good spiritual, emotional, and physical health.

We need to find time and space to practice self-care and make ourselves happy and fulfilled with meaningful and enjoyable activities such as physical exercise, reading, listening to music, dancing, being involved with social activities and volunteer work, and finding enough time for friends and family.

Incorporating self-care and meaningful activities into our lives is, in fact, crucial for overall well-being and happiness.

There are ways to find time and space for these activities while balancing other responsibilities:

- *Prioritize and schedule.* Make self-care a priority by scheduling specific times for these activities in your calendar. Treat them as important appointments that you can't miss.

- *Manage your time.* Evaluate your daily routine and identify pockets of time that can be dedicated to self-care. Cut down on less productive activities or delegate tasks when possible.

- *Set boundaries.* Learn to say no to commitments that don't align with your self-care goals. Setting boundaries helps protect your time and energy.

- *Create morning and evening routines.* Incorporate self-care activities into your morning and evening routines. This can set a positive tone for your day and help you unwind in the evening.

- *Multitask*. Combine activities when possible. For instance, you can listen to music or an audiobook while exercising or doing household chores.

- *Make time for family and friends*. Involve your loved ones in your self-care activities. Go for a walk or exercise together, have a family movie night, or cook a healthy meal as a group.

- *Pursue social activities*. Participate in social activities that align with your interests. This way, you can enjoy yourself while also building connections.

- *Find meaningful volunteer work*. Find volunteer opportunities that resonate with you. Even a few hours a month can make a significant impact and bring a sense of fulfillment.

- *Take mindful breaks*. Incorporate short breaks throughout your day for relaxation or a quick self-care activity. These breaks can boost your mood and productivity.

- *Batch tasks*. Group similar tasks together to make better use of your time and reduce transitions between different activities.

- *Limit screen time*. Cut down on excessive screen time, especially when it doesn't contribute to your well-being. Allocate that time to activities that nurture you.

- *Adapt to changes*. Life can be unpredictable. Be adaptable and willing to adjust your schedule as needed, while still making self-care a priority.

- *Strive for quality over quantity*. Focus on the quality of the time you spend on self-care rather than the quantity. A few minutes of genuine, focused self-care can have a powerful impact.

- *Claim personal space*. Designate a specific area in your home as a personal space for relaxation, reading, or creative activities.

Remember that self-care is not a luxury, but a necessity to build a healthy and fulfilling life.

By making intentional choices and managing your time effectively, you can create a balanced routine that allows you to enjoy meaningful activities and connect with loved ones while meeting other commitments.

Strategies to Mitigate Stress and Slow Aging

Mindfulness and Meditation: Practices like mindfulness meditation can reduce stress levels and improve overall well-being.

Regular Exercise: Physical activity helps manage stress and has numerous health benefits.

Healthy Diet: Eating a balanced diet rich in antioxidants and anti-inflammatory foods can help combat the effects of stress.

Adequate Sleep: Prioritizing good sleep hygiene can improve stress resilience.

Social Connections: Maintaining strong social ties and seeking support can buffer against stress.

By managing stress effectively, it is possible to slow down the aging process and promote overall health and longevity.

POSITIVE AGING STARTS DURING CHILDHOOD

The aging process is a natural part of life that begins from the moment we are born.

While we can't stop the passage of time, we can certainly influence how we age and the quality of our later years through making healthy choices and creating good habits.

This is particularly important for children, as the foundation for a healthy life is often laid during their early years.

Parents, caregivers, and healthcare providers would do well to teach young people how to take the best care of developing bodies and minds.

Here are some key points to consider:

- *Promote a healthy lifestyle.* Encouraging a healthy lifestyle from a young age is crucial. This includes promoting regular physical activity, a balanced diet rich in nutrients, proper hydration, and adequate sleep.

- *Limit inflammatory factors.* Inflammatory processes in the body are associated with various age-related diseases. Reducing exposure to inflammatory factors such as eating unhealthy foods and exposure to food preservatives, food and textile dyes, excessive stress, and environmental toxins can have a positive impact on long-term health.

- *Prevent obesity.* Childhood obesity can lead to several health issues later in life due to the various physiological, psychological, and social effects it has on the body and mind. Here are some key health issues that can arise from childhood obesity:

  - Cardiovascular Diseases

    Obesity in childhood is linked to increased risk factors for cardiovascular diseases, including hypertension (high blood pressure), dyslipidemia (abnormal cholesterol levels), and atherosclerosis (hardening of the arteries).

- Type 2 Diabetes,

    Obesity significantly increases the risk of developing insulin resistance, which can lead to type 2 diabetes. Children with obesity are more likely to become adults with diabetes.

- Musculoskeletal Problems

    Excess weight can put undue stress on bones and joints, leading to conditions like osteoarthritis and other orthopedic issues, including joint pain and musculoskeletal discomfort.

- Respiratory Issues

    Obesity is associated with sleep apnea, asthma, and other respiratory problems due to the excess weight on the chest and abdomen, which can hinder normal breathing patterns.

- Liver Disease

    Non-alcoholic fatty liver disease (NAFLD) is common in obese children, leading to liver inflammation and scarring, which can progress to more severe liver conditions in adulthood.

- Mental Health Disorders

    Children with obesity are at higher risk for mental health issues such as depression, anxiety, and low self-esteem due to stigma, bullying, and body image issues.

- Reproductive Issues

    Obesity can lead to hormonal imbalances that affect puberty and reproductive health. In females, this can result in conditions like polycystic ovary syndrome (PCOS).

- Metabolic Syndrome

    A cluster of conditions include increased blood pressure, high blood sugar levels, excess body fat around the waist, and abnormal cholesterol levels, which together increase the risk of heart disease, stroke, and diabetes.

- Cancer

    Obesity increases the risk of developing certain types of cancer later in life, including breast, colon, and endometrial (uterine) cancer.

- Impact on Quality of Life

    The combination of physical and psychological health issues can lead to a reduced quality of life, affecting social interactions, educational attainment, and overall well-being.

Addressing childhood obesity through proper nutrition, physical activity, and behavioral changes is essential to mitigate these long-term health risks and promote a healthier future for children.

- *Prioritize education.* Teach children about the importance of their choices and how they can impact their future health. Providing them with the knowledge and tools to make informed decisions can empower them to lead healthier lives.

- *Model good choices.* Children often learn by example. Being a positive role model by practicing healthy habits yourself can influence them to adopt similar behaviors.

- *Schedule regular check-ups.* Schedule regular medical and dental check-ups for children to monitor their growth, development, and overall health. Early detection of any potential issues can lead to timely interventions.

- *Promote mental and emotional well-being.* Addressing mental and emotional well-being is as important as physical health. Encourage open communication, emotional expression, and teach coping mechanisms to manage stress.

- *Teach hygiene and safety.* Educate children about proper hygiene practices and safety measures to reduce the risk of infections and accidents.

- *Limit screen time.* Excessive screen time can lead to a sedentary lifestyle, which is detrimental to health. Set limits on screen time and encourage outdoor activities and social interactions.

- *Encourage curiosity and learning.* Foster a love for learning, exploration, and creativity. Engaging in new experiences and challenges can contribute to cognitive health and well-being.

- *Forge healthy relationships.* Teach children about the importance of healthy relationships, both with themselves and with others. Building strong social connections and a positive self-image can contribute to overall well-being.

- *Promote sexual education.* Promoting sexual education in children is essential for their overall well-being, helping them make informed decisions, fostering healthy relationships, and ensuring their safety.

Environmental Factors

Exposure to environmental toxins and chemicals can have significant effects on brain development and potentially contribute to mental and emotional issues in children.

More information is as follows:

- *Neurodevelopmental effects.* Research has shown that exposure to certain environmental pollutants, such as heavy metals (lead, mercury), pesticides, and air pollutants, can interfere with the normal development of the nervous system, including the brain. This interference can potentially lead to cognitive and behavioral impairments in children, which may have implications later in life.

- *Air pollution and autism.* Several studies have suggested a possible association between air pollution and an increased risk of neurodevelopmental disorders, including autism spectrum disorder (ASD). While the exact mechanisms are not fully understood, it's believed that exposure to certain pollutants during critical periods of brain development could contribute to the development of ASD and other neurodevelopmental conditions.

- *Intrauterine exposure.* Emerging evidence indicates that exposure to air pollution during pregnancy, particularly in the early stages, may have a greater impact on neurodevelopment compared to exposure after birth. The developing fetal brain is vulnerable to environmental insults, and prenatal exposure to pollutants could potentially affect brain structure and function.

- *Oxidative stress and inflammation.* Some researchers hypothesize that environmental toxins, including air pollutants, may trigger oxidative stress and inflammation in the developing brain, which could contribute to neurodevelopmental issues.

- *Preventive measures.* To mitigate the potential risks associated with environmental toxins, efforts should be made to reduce exposure. This includes advocating for policies that improve air quality, reducing exposure to harmful chemicals in household products, promoting a healthy diet rich in antioxidants, and avoiding exposure to known toxins during pregnancy.

- *Public awareness and policy.* Raising awareness about the potential risks of environmental toxins and advocating for stricter regulations on pollution and chemical exposure are important steps in protecting children's brain development and overall health.

Research suggests associations between environmental factors and neurodevelopmental issues, but the exact causal relationships are complex and often require further investigation.

Protecting children from environmental toxins is a shared responsibility involving individuals, communities, and governments working together to create healthier environments for future generations.

ANTI-AGING SUPPLEMENTS

Aging is the natural process of cumulative stress and wear and tear on the body. Fortunately, supplements can be helpful in minimizing the impact of oxidative stress while enhancing the body's ability to eliminate toxins, heavy metals, and waste.

Some of these supplements behave as antioxidants:

- *Vitamins.* Vitamin C, vitamin E, and beta-carotene (a precursor of vitamin A) are examples of antioxidant vitamins that can help protect cells from oxidative damage.

- *Minerals.* Selenium and zinc are minerals that play roles as antioxidants in the body.

- *Phytochemicals.* These are naturally occurring compounds found in plants that often have antioxidant properties. Examples include flavonoids, polyphenols, and resveratrol.

- *Enzymes.* Some enzymes in the body, such as superoxide dismutase and glutathione peroxidase, have antioxidant functions.

Glutathione

Glutathione is a powerful antioxidant and plays many other roles in the optimal functioning of our body.

It is a tripeptide molecule composed of three amino acids: cysteine, glycine, and glutamic acid. Glutathione is naturally produced by the body and is found in virtually every cell. It also supports the function of other antioxidants, such as vitamin C and vitamin E, by recycling them and maintaining their active forms.

Glutathione plays additional important roles in the body, such as supporting the immune system, aiding detoxification processes, and contributing to DNA synthesis and repair.

Various factors such as aging, poor diet, stress, environmental toxins, and certain medical conditions can lead to decreased levels of glutathione. Low levels of glutathione have been linked to the development of macular degeneration. This has led to interest in using glutathione supplements or treatments to potentially enhance antioxidant defenses and overall health.

How do we naturally increase our endogenous production of GSH (Glutathione) in the body? Increasing the endogenous production GSH in the body can be achieved through various natural methods.

Here are some effective strategies:

Dietary Intake

- *Sulfur-rich foods.* Sulfur is a key component of glutathione. Foods rich in sulfur include garlic, onions, cruciferous vegetables such as broccoli, cauliflower, Brussels sprouts, and kale, and asparagus.

- *Whey protein.* This contains cysteine, which is a precursor to glutathione. Ensure it is of high quality and free from added sugars and artificial ingredients.

- *Antioxidant-rich foods.* Consuming foods high in vitamins C and E, such as fruits; oranges, strawberries, and kiwi, and vegetables; bell peppers and spinach can help regenerate glutathione.

- *Selenium-rich foods.* Selenium is a cofactor for the enzyme glutathione peroxidase. Brazil nuts, sunflower seeds, and mushrooms are good sources.

Supplements

- *N-Acetylcysteine (NAC).* This supplement provides cysteine, a direct precursor to glutathione.

- *Alpha-lipoic acid.* This antioxidant helps to regenerate glutathione and supports mitochondrial function.

- *Milk thistle.* This contains silymarin, which may support liver health and boost glutathione production.

- *Vitamins C and E.* These vitamins can help maintain glutathione levels in the body.

Lifestyle Factors

- *Regular exercise.* Moderate-intensity exercise can boost antioxidant defenses, including glutathione levels. Both aerobic exercise and resistance training are beneficial.

- *Adequate sleep.* Proper rest supports overall health and the body's ability to produce antioxidants, including glutathione.

- *Stress management.* Chronic stress can deplete glutathione levels. Practices such as meditation, yoga, and deep-breathing exercises can help manage stress.

Avoiding Toxins

- *Minimize exposure to environmental toxins.* Reducing exposure to pollutants, chemicals, and heavy metals can help preserve glutathione levels.

- *Avoid smoking and excessive alcohol consumption.* These habits can deplete glutathione and other antioxidants.

Hydration

- *Stay well-hydrated.* Adequate water intake is essential for all cellular functions, including the production of glutathione.

By incorporating these dietary, supplemental, and lifestyle changes, you can naturally boost your body's production of glutathione, enhancing your overall antioxidant defense system.

While antioxidants are important for maintaining cellular health and potentially reducing the impact of oxidative stress, the relationship between antioxidant supplementation and longevity or age-related diseases is still an area of active research and debate.

Some studies have shown potential benefits of antioxidants in certain contexts, while others have raised concerns about the potential for excessive antioxidant supplementation to interfere with natural cellular processes. Moreover, the effectiveness of antioxidant supplements can vary based on factors such as the specific antioxidant, its dosage, the individual's overall health status, and the presence of other nutrients and compounds that interact with antioxidants.

As with any supplementation, it's important to approach it with caution and under the guidance of a healthcare professional.

Balanced and varied diets rich in fruits, vegetables, and other nutrient-dense foods remain one of the best strategies for obtaining a wide range of antioxidants and supporting overall health as you age.

CONCLUSION

In conclusion, this publication seeks to empower patients with scientific knowledge to make informed decisions about their health, leading to positive lifestyle changes.

The psychological impact of an HPV diagnosis is significant, causing anxiety and relationship concerns. As we age, clearing the virus becomes less likely due to slower tissue turnover. Moreover, caring for HPV patients has a socioeconomic impact, with high healthcare costs, especially for cancer treatment. However, universal HPV vaccination can prevent these diseases, reduce healthcare costs, and improve patients' quality of life. This publication aims to raise awareness about HPV and promote overall health.

I am a firm believer in empowering people through education. Ignorance and prejudice are the sources of many ailments of our society. The importance of knowledge and education in shaping a society and its values cannot be overstated.

Knowledge provides people with the tools to make informed decisions, helping them navigate the complexities of the world. An educated mind can distinguish between right and wrong, fact and fiction, and make choices based on reason rather than impulse.

Proper education teaches individuals to think critically. Critical thinking is the bedrock of a progressive society, allowing people to challenge outdated norms, question authority when needed, and innovate for the betterment of all.

Ignorance often breeds fear, and fear can easily lead to prejudice. When individuals are educated about cultures, religions, histories, and philosophies other than their own, it fosters empathy and understanding. This can significantly reduce prejudiced beliefs and biases.

On a pragmatic level, an educated populace contributes to a nation's economic growth. They can better contribute to the workforce, innovate, and adapt to changing environments.

An educated populace is more likely to be engaged in civic activities, whether that is voting, volunteering, or participating in community projects. This ensures that the voices of the many, rather than the few, guide the direction of society.

Knowledge acts as a shield against manipulation. When people are educated, they are less likely to fall prey to scams, misleading information, or propaganda. Through education, individuals can be introduced to concepts of morality, ethics, and the greater good. This can lead to a more compassionate society where the rights of individuals are respected and mutual respect is a given.

However, while education is a powerful tool, it's essential to remember that it's not just about traditional forms of learning. Education should be holistic, encouraging emotional intelligence, life skills, and practical know-how. Only then can it truly foster well-rounded individuals capable of bringing meaningful societal changes.

A quote widely attributed to Nelson Mandela is "Education is the most powerful weapon which you can use to change the world." I do believe in the positive transformative power of education.

Every individual, regardless of culture or background, seeks happiness and well-being as a foundation for mutual respect and tolerance.

When we approach interactions with the understanding that our shared humanity is greater than our differences, it fosters empathy, reduces prejudices, and promotes peaceful coexistence. Embracing diversity and seeking to understand others enriches our own lives, broadens our perspectives, and builds stronger, more inclusive communities.

At the core of our being, we yearn for connection, belonging, and affection. From familial bonds to societal networks, the feeling of being cherished provides emotional security and well-being. The need to communicate and be understood is essential.

Listening is more than just hearing words; it's about comprehension, empathy, and validation. Every individual craves the liberty to express their thoughts, beliefs, and feelings without fear of judgment or repression.

The desire to coexist peacefully, both with fellow humans and the environment, reflects our innate longing for stability, balance, and sustainability. Recognizing and respecting these universal desires can lead to more inclusive, empathetic, and harmonious societies. It underscores the importance of fostering environments where these needs are met and celebrated.

REFERENCES

Boudreau, M. D., F. A Beland, J. A. Nichols, M. Pogribna. 2013. "Toxicology and Carcinogenesis Studies of a Nondecolorized Whole Leaf Extract of Aloe barbadensis Miller (Aloe vera) in F344/Nrats and B6C3F1 mice (drinking water study). *Natl Toxicol Program Tech Rep Ser.* Aug:(577):1–266.

Braaten and Laufer. 2008. "Human Papillomavirus (HPV), HPV-Related Disease, and the HPV Vaccine." *Reviews in Obstetrics and Gynecology.* Winter; 1(1):2–10. PMID: 18701931; PMCID: PMC2492590.

Camilleri, Michael. 2019. "Leaky gut: mechanisms, measurement and clinical implications in humans." Gut 68:1516–1526. doi. org/10.3390/ijms22147613

Camilleri, Michael. 2021. "What is the leaky gut? Clinical considerations in humans." *Current Opinion in Clinical Nutrition and Metabolic Care.* September. 24(5): 473–482. doi. org/10.1097/MCO.0000000000000778

CDC. 2023. "Cancers Linked With HPV Each Year." www.cdc.gov/cancer/hpv/cases.html

Cox, J. Thomas. 2004. "Liquid-Based Cytology: Evaluation of Effectiveness, Cost-effectiveness, and Application to Present Practice. J Natl Compr Canc Netw. Nov;2(6):597–611. doi. org/10.6004/jnccn.2004.0050.

Dahoud, Wissam, Claire W. Michael, Hamza Gokozan, Amelia K Nakanishi, Aparna Harbhajanka. 2019. "Association of Bacterial Vaginosis and Human Papilloma Virus Infection with Cervical

Squamous Intraepithelial Lesions." *American Journal of Clinical Pathology* 152:2 August. 185–189. doi.org/10.1093/ajcp/aqz021

Fakhry, Carole, Qiang Zhang, Phuc Felix Nguyen-Tan, David Rosenthal, Adel El-Naggar, Adam S. Garden, Denis Soulieres, Andy Trotti, Vilija Avizonis, John Andrew Ridge, Jonathan Harris, Quynh-Thu Le, Maura Gillison. 2014. "Human Papillomavirus and Overall Survival After Progression of Oropharyngeal Squamous Cell Carcinoma." *Journal of Clinical Oncology.* Oct. 20;32(30):3365–73. doi.org/10.1200/JCO.2014.55.1937

Hurtado-Salgado, Erika, Luz Cárdenas- Cárdenas, Jorge Salmerón, Rufino Luna-Gordillo, Eduardo Ortiz-Panozo, Betania Allen-Leigh, Nenetzen Saavedra-Lara, Eduardo L. Franco, Eduardo Lazcano-Ponce. 2021. "Comparative performance of the human papillomavirus test and cytology for primary screening for high-grade cervical intraepithelial neoplasia at the population level." International Journal of Cancer. 150 (2021): 1422–1430. doi.org/10.102/ijc.33905

Kumar, Ramesh and Amit Kumar Singh, Ashutosh Gupta, Anupam Bishayee, Abhay K. Pandy. 2019. "Therapeutic potential of Aloe vera—A miracle gift of nature." *Phytomedicine.* Vol. 60, July. 152996. doi.org/10.1016/j.phymed.2019.152996

Lewis, Rayleen M., Jean-Francois Laprise, Julia W. Gargano, Elizabeth R. Unger, Troy D. Querec, Harrell W. Chesson, Marc Brisson, Lauri E. Markowitz. 2021. "Estimated Prevalence and Incidence of Disease-Associated Human Papillomavirus Types Among 15- to 59-Year-Olds in the United States." Sex Transm Dis. Apr 1;48(4):273–277. doi.org/10.1097/OLQ.0000000000001356.

Liu, Yang, Jing Liao, Xiaojia Yi, Zhengmei Pan, Chunyi Sun, Hoglin Zhou, Yushi Meng. 2022. "Diagnostic value of colposcopy in patients with cytology-negative and HR-HPV-positive cervical lesions." *Arch Gynecol Obstet* 306, 1161–1169. doi.org/10.1007/s00404-022-06415-5

Massad, L. Stewart, Mark H. Einstein, Warner K. Huh, Hormuzd A. Katki, Walter K. Kinney, Mark Schiffman, Diane Solomon, Nicolas Wentzensen, Herschel W. Lawson. 2013. "2012 Updated Consensus Guidelines for the Management of Abnormal Cervical Cancer Screening Tests and Cancer Precursors." *Journal of Lower Genital Tract Disease*. 17(5 Suppl 1), S1–S27. doi.org/10.1097/AOG.0b013e3182883a34

McCullough, Marjorie L., Emilie S. Zoltick, Stephanie J. Weinstein, Veronika Fedirko, Molin Wang, Nancy R. Cook, A. Heather Eliassen, Anne Zeleniuch-Jacquotte, Claudia Agnoli, Demetrius Albanes, Matthew J. Barnett, Julie E. Buring, Peter T. Campbell, Tess V. Clendenen, Neal D. Freedman, Susan M. Gapsturf, Edward L. Giovannucci, Gary G. Goodman, Christopher A. Haiman, Gloria Y. F. Ho, Ronald L. Horst, Tao Hou, Wen-Yi Huang, Mazda Jenab, Michael E. Jones, Corinne E. Joshu, Vittorio Krogh, I-Min Lee, Jung Eun Lee, Satu Männistö, Loic Le Marchand, Alison M. Mondul, Marian L. Neuhouser, Elizabeth A. Platz, Mark P. Purdue, Elio Riboli, Trude Eid Robsahm, Thomas E. Rohan, Shizuka Sasazuki, Minouk J. Schoemaker, Sabina Sieri, Meir J. Stampfer, Anthony J Swerdlow, Cynthia A Thomson, Steinar Tretli, Schoichiro Tsugane, Giske Ursin, Kala Visvanathan, Kami K. WhiteKana Wu, Shiaw-Shyuan Yaun, Xuehong Zhang, Walter C. Willett, Mitchel H. Gail, Regina G. Ziegler, Stephanie A. Smith-Warner. 2019. "Circulating Vitamin D and Colorectal Cancer Risk: An International Pooling Project of 17 Cohorts." *J Natl Cancer Inst*. Feb 1;111(2):158-169. doi.org/10.1093/jnci/djy087

Moscicki, Anna-Barbara, Stephen Shiboski, Jeannette Broering, Kimberly Powell, Lisa Clayton, Naomi Jay, Teresa M. Darragh, Robert Brescia, Saul Kanowitz, Susanna B. Miller, Joanna Stone, Evelyn Hanson, Joel Palefsky. 1998. "The Natural History of Human Papillomavirus Infection as Measured by Repeated DNA Testing in Adolescent and Young Women." *Journal Pediatrics*. February 132:2. 277–284. doi.org/10.1016/S0022-3476(98)70445-7

Najib, Fatemeh Sadat, Masooumeh Hashemi, Zahra Shiravani, Tahereh Poordast, Sanam Sharifi, Elham Askary. 2020. "Diagnostic accuracy of cervical Pap smear and colposcopy in detecting premalignant and malignant lesions of the cervix." *Indian J Surg. Onc.* Sept; 11:2 453–458. doi.org/10.1007/s13193-020-01118-2

Omranipour, Ramesh, Ali Kazemian, Sadaf Alipour, Masoume Najafi, Mansour Alidoosti, Mitra Navid, Afsaneh Alikhassi, Nasrin Ahmadinejad, Khojasteh Bagheri, Shahrzad Izadi. 2016. "Comparison of the Accuracy of Thermography and Mammography in the Detection of Breast Cancer." *Breast Care* (2016) 11(4): 260–264. doi.org/10.1159/000448347

Pingali, Cassandra, David Yankey, Laurie D. Elam-Evans, Lauri E. Markowitz, Charnetta L. Williams, Benjamin Fredua, Lucy A. McNamara, Shannon Stokley, James A. Singleton. 2021. "National, Regional, State, and Selected Local Area Vaccination Coverage Among Adolescents Aged 13–17 Years—United States, 2020." *MMWR Morb Mortal Wkly Rep* 2021; 70:1183–1190. doi.org/10.15585/mmwr.mm7035a1

Proma, Paul, Anne Hammer, Anne F. Rositch, Anne E. Burke, Raphael P. Visidi, Michelle I. Silver, Nicole Campos, Ada O. Youk, Patti E. Gravitt. 2021. "Rates of New Human

Papillomavirus Detection and Loss of Detection in Middle-aged Women by Recent and Past Sexual Behavior." The Journal of Infectious Diseases, Volume 223, Issue 8, 15 April 2021, Pages 1423–1432. doi.org/10.1093/infdis/jiaa557

Radosevich, James. 2019. *HPV and Cancer*. Springer.

Rossi, Emma C. 2018. "Vaginal intraepithelial neoplasia: What to do when dysplasia persists after hysterectomy." MDedge. September 18. mdedge.com/obgyn/article/175084/gynecologic-cancer/vaginal-intraepithelial-neoplasia-what-do-when-dysplasia

Supramanya, Deepthi and Petros D. Grivas. 2008. "HPV and Cervical Cancer: Updates on an Established Relationship." Postgrad Med. 2008 Nov;120(4):7–13. doi.org/10.3810/pgm.2008.11.1928

Swiderska-Kiec, Joanna, Krzysztof Czajkowski, Julia Zareba-S. 2020. "Comparison of HPV Testing and Colposcopy in Detecting Cervical Dysplasia in Patients with Cytological Abnormalities." *In Vivo*. May, 34:3 1307–1315. doi.org/10.21873/invivo.11906

Usuda, Haruki, Okamoto Tkayuki, Koichiro Wada. 2021. "Leaky Gut: Effect of Dietary Fiber and Fats on Microbiome and Intestinal Barrier." *Int. J. Mol. Sci.* 22(14), 7613; doi.org/10.3390/ijms22147613

Van Dyne E. A., S. J. Henley, M. Saraiya, C. C. Thomas, L. E. Markowitz, V. B. Benard. 2018. "Trends in Human Papillomavirus–Associated Cancers—United States, 1999–2015." *MMWR Morb Mortal Wkly Rep* 67:918–924. doi.org/10.15585/mmwr.mm6733a2.

NUMBERED REFERENCE LIST

1) https://www.cdc.gov/cancer/hpv/cases.html

2) (Braaten and Laufer, 2008)

3) (James Radosevich, Ph.D. "HPV and cancer" Springer, 2012)

4) https://www.cdc.gov/vaccines/vpd/hpv/hcp/safety-effectiveness.html

5) https://medlineplus.gov/vaginitis.html

6) https://www.ncbi.nlm.nih.gov/books/NBK459216

7) (Dahoud, et al. 2019)

8) https://pmc.ncbi.nlm.nih.gov/articles/PMC5694177

9) https://pmc.ncbi.nlm.nih.gov/articles/PMC3889747

10) https://www.cdc.gov/cancer/hpv/diagnosis-by-age.html

11) https://www.cdc.gov/cancer/hpv/diagnosis-by-age.html

12) https://screening.iarc.fr/atlasHPV.php

13) https://pmc.ncbi.nlm.nih.gov/articles/PMC7855977/#B10

14) https://pmc.ncbi.nlm.nih.gov/articles/PMC7855977/#B11

(15) https://www.sciencedirect.com/science/article/pii/0091743589900017

16) HPV and Cervical Cancer: Updates on an Established Relationship: Postgraduate Medicine: Vol 120, No 4

17) https://onlinelibrary.wiley.com/doi/10.1111/ijd.13697

Empower Your Health

18) (Souza, et al. 2007, 2010; Gillison, et al. 2008; Heck, et al 2010, Smith, et al. 2004)

19) https://pmc.ncbi.nlm.nih.gov/articles/PMC10047250

20) (Bonnez and Reichman, 2010; CDC, 2010a)

21) https://www.cdc.gov/sti/media/images/SPICE-prevalence-vs-incidence.png

22) https://pubmed.ncbi.nlm.nih.gov/27345585

23) https://ajcn.nutrition.org/article/S0002-9165(22)03668-1/fulltext

24) https://www.annalsofoncology.org/article/S0923-7534(21)01993-1/fulltext

25) https://pubmed.ncbi.nlm.nih.gov/33553987

26) https://pmc.ncbi.nlm.nih.gov/articles/PMC5088670

27) https://pubmed.ncbi.nlm.nih.gov/21223574

28) https://www.sleephealth.org

About The Author

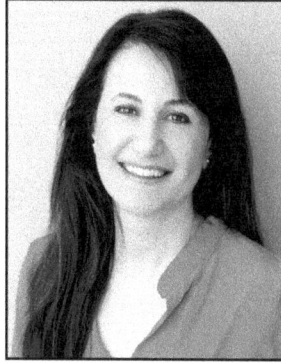

Lucia Cagnes, MD, earned her medical degree from the University of Palermo Medical School in Italy, where she also attained board certification in Obstetrics and Gynecology. She then completed her full OB/GYN training in the United States, becoming board certified here in 1999. Over four decades of clinical practice and personal interactions, Dr. Cagnes witnessed firsthand the serious health implications associated with HPV. Motivated by these experiences, she pursued an extensive review of scientific evidence, organizing key findings that she now shares with her patients, loved ones, and readers. Dr. Cagnes currently practices medicine and resides in Massachusetts.

www.ingramcontent.com/pod-product-compliance
Lightning Source LLC
Chambersburg PA
CBHW062128020426
42335CB00013B/1138